OFFICE

PROCEDURES

OFFICE

PROCEDURES

THOMAS J. ZUBER, MD

Program Director in Family Medicine
Saginaw Cooperative Hospitals
Saginaw, Michigan
Associate Professor
Michigan State University
Director, Dermatology Clinic
Aleda E. Lutz
VA Medical Center
Saginaw, Michigan

Series Medical Editor
RICHARD SADOVSKY, MD, MS
Associate Professor of Family Medicine
State University of New York
  Health Science Center
Brooklyn, New York

Williams & Wilkins
A WAVERLY COMPANY
BALTIMORE ¥ PHILADELPHIA ¥ LONDON ¥ PARIS ¥ BANGKOK
HONG KONG ¥ MUNICH ¥ SYDNEY ¥ TOKYO ¥ WROCLAW

Editor: Jonathan W. Pine, Jr.
Development Editor: Robert Newman, Co Medica, Inc
Project Manager, AAFP: Leigh McKinney
Managing Editor: Molly L. Mullen
Marketing Manager: Daniell Griffin
Production Editor: Jennifer D. Weir

Copyright © 1999 Williams & Wilkins

351 West Camden Street
Baltimore, Maryland 21201-2436 USA

Rose Tree Corporate Center
1400 North Providence Road
Building II, Suite 5025
Media, Pennsylvania 19063-2043 USA

Printed in the United States of America

Library of Congress Cataloging-in-Publication Data

Zuber, Thomas J.
    Office procedures/Thomas J. Zuber.
    (The Academy collection—quick reference guides for family physicians)
    At head of title: American Academy of Family Physicians.
    Includes bibliographical references and index.
    ISBN 0-683-30424-0
    1. Ambulatory surgery. 2. Family medicine. I. American Academy of Family Physicians. II. Title. III. Series.
    [DNLM: 1. Ambulatory Surgical Procedures—methods. 2. Biopsy—methods. 3. Family Practice—methods. WO 192 Z93 1998]
    RD110.Z83   1998
    617'.024—dc21
    DNLM/DLC
    for Library of Congress   98-22560
                                                  CIP

The publishers have made every effort to trace the copyright holders for borrowed material. If they have inadvertently overlooked any, they will be pleased to make the necessary arrangements at the first opportunity.

To purchase additional copies of this book, call our customer service department at **(800) 638-0672** or fax orders to **(800) 447-8438.** For other book services, including chapter reprints and large quantity sales, ask for the Special Sales department.

Canadian customers should call **(800) 665-1148,** or fax **(800) 665-0103.** For all other calls originating outside of the United States, please call **(410) 528-4223** or fax us at **(410) 528-8550.**

Visit *Williams & Wilkins* on the *Internet:* http://www.wwilkins.com or contact our customer service department at **custserv@wwilkins.com.** Williams & Wilkins customer service representatives are available from 8:30 am to 6:00 pm, EST, Monday through Friday, for telephone access.

99 00 01 02 03
1 2 3 4 5 6 7 8 9 10

This book has required many long hours for completion. I want to dedicate it to those who sacrificed so much for its completion: Julie, Laura, TJ, and Andrew. I also acknowledge the encouragement of those physicians who have fought for the place of procedures in family medicine.

Thomas J. Zuber

SERIES INTRODUCTION

Family practice is a unique clinical specialty encompassing a philosophy of care rather than a modality of care provided to a specific segment of the population. This philosophy of providing longitudinal care for persons of all ages in the complete context of their physical, emotional, and social environments was modeled by general practitioners, the parents of our modern specialty. To provide this kind of care, the family physician needs a broad knowledge base, appropriate evaluation tools, effective interventions, and patient education.

The knowledge base needed by a family physician is extraordinarily large. The American Academy of Family Physicians and other organizations provide clinical education through conferences and journals. Individual family physicians have written journal articles about a specific clinical topic or have tried to cover the broad knowledge base of family medicine in a single volume. The former are helpful, but may cover only a narrow segment of medicine, while the latter may not provide the depth needed to be useful in actual patient care.

The Academy Collection: Quick Reference Guides for Family Physicians is a series of books designed to assist family physicians with the broad knowledge base unique to our specialty. The books in this series have all been written by practicing family physicians who have special interest in the topics, and the chapters have been formatted to provide easy access to information needed at varying stages in the physician-patient encounter. Each volume is unique because each author has personalized the volume and provided a unique family physician perspective.

This series is not meant to be a final reference for the family physician who seeks a comprehensive text. The series also does not cover every topic that may be encountered by the family physician. The series does offer, in a depth determined appropriate by the authors, the information needed by the physician to handle the majority of patient encounters. The series also provides information to make patient care a combined doctor-patient effort. Specific patient education materials have been included where appropriate. Readers can contact the American Academy of Family Physicians Foundation for other resources.

The topics selected for **The Academy Collection** were chosen based on what family physicians said they needed. The first group of books covers office procedures, conditions of aging, and some of the most challenging diagnoses seen in family practice. Future books in the series will address musculoskeletal problems, occupational/environmental medicine, skin conditions, children's health, and gastrointestinal problems.

I welcome your comments. Please contact me at the American Academy of Family Physicians with your suggestions. This collection is meant to be useful to you and your patients.

Richard Sadovsky, MD, MS
Series Editor
The Academy Collection
c/o AAFP, 8880 Ward Parkway
Kansas City, MO 64116
e-mail: academycollection@aafp.org

CONTENTS

··

SECTION III

DIAGNOSTIC AND THERAPEUTIC PROCEDURES 157

INTRODUCTION

I am a firm believer in the value to patients and the health care system of family physicians performing diagnostic and therapeutic office procedures. Family physicians, like other medical specialists, can easily learn the specific mechanical techniques for any procedure. Family physicians desire to provide these services with the same high quality they provide through their other services. Patients benefit from having procedures performed in the familiar, and often less-expensive, environment of their family physician's office. Continuity of care is enhanced when patients stay in their physician's office and have less fragmentation of care by multiple physician referrals.

When I was asked to author this book, my initial response was that I did not want to repeat the fine work that already exists in other procedural medicine textbooks; however, there has been a void of practical resources for physicians who wish to incorporate procedural services into their offices. My years of teaching procedural medicine nationally have uncovered frequent problems that physicians have in setting up systems to make their services flow smoothly. It is for these physicians that this book is written. Although the mechanics of the procedures are discussed here, it is the procedure set-up, review of pitfalls and complications, follow-up instructions, equipment ordering information, and billing instructions that make this procedural resource stand out.

A separate book has been created to accompany this textbook, with patient education sheets, nursing instruction sheets, informed consent forms, and procedure recording forms. These sheets can be copied right onto a physician's office letterhead, thereby personalizing them. I believe this additional text will save physicians time, streamline their patient education efforts, and make the incorporation of procedural services easier. I also hope that the quality of patient services can be enhanced by the materials that are contained in both texts.

How to Use This Book

The main chapters include a description of the procedure, as performed in my office. There are many ways to perform each procedure. I have selected techniques based on years of experience, patient feedback, and complications reported in the medical literature. The rationale for a specific technique is included in some chapters. In some cases, alternative procedure choices are also listed.

If the reader wishes to use my technique, the materials and equipment I use are included. It is not my intention to endorse any single company's products or materials. I am not paid by any of these companies, nor do I have any formal contractual ties to them; however, physicians frequently ask which equipment I select. When a particular piece of equipment is useful in my technique, that equipment is listed. I have tried to list as many different manufacturers as possible. If several endoscopes are of similar cost and quality, I may list a particular company's endoscope because that manufacturer has not been listed in other parts of the book.

The procedure set-up section of each chapter is designed to help offices prepare efficiently for office surgical procedures. The list of materials for each procedure can be placed into a notebook for easy nursing access. Some materials may be added or deleted by a particular office, depending on the physician's preference.

A section on procedure pitfalls is included in most chapters. These pitfalls include mistakes I have witnessed or heard about over the years. Novice physicians in any procedure often stumble over similar problems. It is hoped that this section will aid physicians in avoiding these problem areas. Some chapters also list clinical situations that are amenable and not amenable to the technique.

Some chapters include special information, such as indications or contraindications for a particular procedure. Drawings were included where they were felt to enhance understanding. The chapter on thoracentesis includes information regarding the common results of fluid analysis of exudates and transudates. The chapter on nasolaryngoscopy includes a brief listing of the common anatomic areas visualized. It is hoped that these additional sections will enhance the physician's understanding and appropriate use of each procedure.

A brief section is included regarding the training of physicians in each procedure. This book is in no way intended to replace hands-on, supervised training. How much training is required is a difficult area to address. The American Academy of Family Physicians has attempted to provide guidance to physicians in the necessary training for many areas of procedural medicine. Proper training and competency are individual issues for every physician. Although some physicians can competently perform chalazion removal after just three precepted procedures, other physicians may require more than 30 procedures before they feel comfortable with the technique and can perform the procedure unassisted. I urge the reader not to latch on to a specific number of procedures as an indicator of competency. Rather, competency comes from reading, attending formal courses, watching others performing the technique, practicing manual skills, and precepted patient experiences.

A section on follow-up instructions for each procedure has been included. This section includes actions for the physician after obtaining the most common pathology results for a particular procedure. For instance, the therapeutic options available for managing CIN 1 on colposcopic biopsy are discussed in the colposcopy chapter. I also list the follow-up visits to schedule after the LEEP procedure.

Setting up a properly functioning office includes the proper coding and billing of procedural services to third-party payers. Office reporting systems frequently rely on office personnel to recreate the services performed in the surgical room. I urge physicians to take an active role in coding their services. Some basic coding information related to these procedures is included in each chapter. Included with the CPT codes are the relative values assigned to each service by the Health Care Services Administration for 1998 (1). Relative value units can be used to set fees for a particular service (2). Also included are the average 50th percentile fees for these services in 1997 (3). Knowing these average charges for a particular service can help physicians communicate with patients who have been told that the physician's charge exceeds the insurance company's allowable limit. Physicians can reassure patients that they are not overbilling, but that the insurance company may be underpaying.

A list of about 10 important literature resources is included with each chapter to encourage physicians to look at other printed materials. For some procedures, such as nasolaryngoscopy, a list of additional educational videotapes is included. The best physicians are lifelong students, and all medical providers should constantly seek ways to improve their performance.

For those interested, a supplemental book of procedural office forms is available as a companion to this book. Included in this supplement are patient education sheets, informed consent forms, nursing instructions, and procedure recording sheets.

Thomas T. Zuber, MD

REFERENCES

1. Physicians' Current Procedural Terminology (CPT 1998). Chicago: American Medical Association, 1998.

2. Department of Health and Human Services, Health Care Financing Administration. Medicare program: revisions to payment policies and adjustments to the relative value units under the physician fee schedule for calendar year 1998. Federal Register 42 CFR parts 400, 405, 410, 411 and 414. October 31, 1997;62(211):59048-59260.

3. 1998 Physicians' Fee Reference. West Allis, WI: Yale Wasserman, DMD, Medical Publishers, 1998.

DIAGNOSTIC PROCEDURES

CHAPTER 1

....

Colposcopy

Colposcopy is the magnified examination of the cervix and female genital tract, using a special microscope called a colposcope. Colposcopy, combined with directed biopsies and endocervical curettage, has become the accepted method of evaluation of patients with an abnormal Pap smear (Table 1.1). Colposcopic biopsies have supplanted the blind or "four-quadrant" biopsy techniques and yield improved diagnostic accuracy regarding the extent of cervical disease. Colposcopy is commonly used to triage patients into conservative or surgical management strategies.

A major area of focus during colposcopy is the squamocolumnar junction (SCJ), the interface of the squamous mucosa of the ectocervix with the columnar mucosa of the endocervical canal. Because the vast majority of cervical cancers develop at or adjacent to the SCJ, visualization of the complete junction is important for the colposcopy procedure to be considered adequate. The SCJ constantly changes throughout the woman's reproductive years, often extending outward after puberty, and retracting inside the endocervical canal after menopause.

In the past, more than 90% of all cervical cancers were squamous cell carcinoma (SCC). However, in the past two decades, the incidence of adenocarcinoma has steadily increased. The natural history of adenocarcinoma appears to be different than that of SCC, and adenocarcinoma may develop without the precursor stages seen with squamous cancers. Patients exhibiting even mild endocervical changes should be evaluated colposcopically, and followed closely. Mild squamous cell changes, such as atypia, may not require immediate triage to colposcopy. Many experts recommend that two Pap smears be reported with atypical squamous cells of undetermined significance (ASCUS) before the patient is considered for colposcopy.

Squamous dysplasia is considered to be a premalignant transformation of the cervical tissues, due in part to the human papillomavirus (HPV). Dysplasia was previously considered to be a continuum from mild to moderate to severe change. It is now understood that mild dysplasia is very similar to atypical cellular change, and probably represents more of a tissue response to HPV than a true premalignant change. Moderate and severe dysplasia are considered to be high-grade squamous intraepithelial lesions, and probably represent premalignant change. High-grade changes are usually treated with

TABLE 1.1.   Indications for Colposcopy

Pap smear suggesting dysplasia or cancer
Pap smear suggesting any adenomatous abnormality (including atypia)
Two Pap smears reporting atypical squamous cells of undetermined significance (ASCUS)
Suspicious visible or palpable lesion of the cervix or genital tract
Patients with a history of intrauterine diethylstilbestrol exposure
Follow up of a patient with a cervix that has previously been surgically treated
Follow up of a patient with persisting abnormal Pap smear
Follow up of a patient previously treated for genital tract cancer

surgical interventions such as loop electrosurgical excision procedure (LEEP) or laser conization.

Disease in the endocervical canal may behave differently than disease on the ectocervix. Mild dysplasia on the ectocervix probably resolves spontaneously in the majority of women, and often does not require surgical intervention. Most experts recommend treatment of mild dysplasia within the canal, as this may have a much more serious prognosis.

Endocervical curettage is considered to be the standard method of evaluating the endocervical canal during colposcopy. The cytobrush can be substituted since it provides a similar specimen, without the discomfort caused by endocervical curettage. While substituting the brush has not been uniformly accepted in the United States, other techniques are being used to reduce discomfort from the procedure. It is often recommended that women take preprocedure ibuprofen (Motrin). Some physicians spray benzocaine (Hurricaine) onto the cervix before performing cervical biopsies.

Several studies have demonstrated the benefits of educating women regarding the colposcopy procedure, the importance of cervical cancer screening, and the value of follow-up visits. To accomplish these goals, patient information sheets can be mailed to patients prior to the visit. A major portion of the colposcopy visit can also be spent educating the patient regarding cervical dysplasia and HPV. Some physicians believe that enhancing the immune system by discontinuing smoking can aid in controlling the changes of HPV. The role of multivitamins with antioxidants may be beneficial, but is as yet unproved.

METHODS AND MATERIALS

Patient Preparation

Ask the patient to undress from the waist down. The patient is given a sheet to cover her waist and legs. The patient is seated on the examination table to talk with the physician.

Equipment
Nonsterile Tray for the Procedure
Place the following items on a nonsterile sheet covering the Mayo stand:

Nonsterile Graves' large vaginal speculum

12 large cotton-tipped swabs

12 small cotton-tipped swabs

2 labeled formalin specimen containers

Acetic acid in a small plastic medicine cup

Monsel's's solution in a small plastic medicine cup

Ring (Foerster) forceps

Tischler cervical biopsy forceps instrument

Endocervical curette (without basket)

Endocervical speculum (if desired)

Wooden toothpicks (for removing biopsy specimens from biopsy instrument)

Cut piece of Telfa pad (½ inch × ½ inch)

Absorbent external pad (to place in the underwear after the procedure)

PROCEDURE DESCRIPTION

1. The patient is placed in the dorsal lithotomy position, with the feet placed in stirrups. The colposcope is turned on, and the instrument is positioned so that the light shines on the vulvar tissues. The vulvar tissues are examined with the naked eye and abnormalities are noted. Some physicians routinely place acetic acid on the vulva and examine the tissues under the colposcope.
2. The speculum is gently inserted, positioning the cervix in the center of the speculum. The cervix and vagina are wiped clear of any mucus or debris. The colposcope is positioned so the cervix is well illuminated, and then the scope is focused on the cervix, initially using low magnification.
3. Acetic acid is applied to the cervix using cotton balls (held in ring forceps) or large cotton-tipped swabs. The acetic acid should be applied to the tissue surface, and not vigorously wiped on, which can cause trauma and bleeding. Leaving the swab adjacent to the cervix for 30 seconds can create good acetic acid effect. If the colposcopic examination is lengthy, a reapplication of acetic acid may be needed every 2 to 5 minutes.

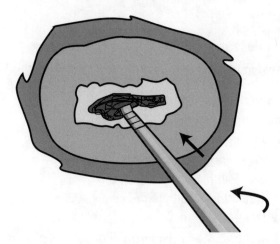

FIGURE 1.1. Endocervical curettage (ECC) is performed with the curette placed inside the canal, and the instrument is vigorously scraped against the endocervical wall while simultaneously turning the instrument through two 360-degree turns. The curette remains in the canal for the entire procedure, and ECC usually takes only 10 to 15 seconds to perform.

4. Areas of acetowhite, vascular change, or surface contour change should be recorded. The most abnormal appearing areas are recorded, and these will be the sites for subsequent biopsy. Higher magnification and the green filter can be used to further evaluate the cervix through the colposcope. The entire extent of the SCJ must be identified in order for the colposcopic evaluation to be considered adequate. Some physicians routinely examine the endocervical canal with an endocervical speculum to look for gross or white lesions that might indicate the need for conization.

5. The endocervical curettage (ECC) is performed to evaluate the cells of the endocervical canal. The ECC is performed by keeping the curette within the canal and scraping all the walls vigorously and circumferentially twice (Figure 1.1). This appears to decrease the chance of inadequate sampling. A well-performed ECC can be performed in 10 to 15 seconds. Some physicians alternately perform this examination with the cytobrush. The brush may be more accurate if it doesn't inadvertently sample cells from the ectocervix. A straw can be used to shield the brush on insertion, and the straw can be withdrawn just before the brush is rotated 180° in the canal. To help with the discomfort and cramping produced by the ECC, patients can take preprocedure ibuprofen. The patient can be encouraged to pant or perform labor breathing during the discomfort of the ECC procedure.

6. The endocervical curette can be swished side to side in the formalin bottle to release the mucus and cellular specimen. Do not bang the front edge of the curette against the specimen container, as this can dull the instrument. Significant cellular sample still remains in the canal mucus. The ring forceps can be used to grasp the mucus without damaging the cervix. The mucus is then squeezed onto a small ½-inch × ½-inch cut piece of Telfa. The Telfa is dropped into the specimen container; then the endocervical cells will be centrifuged away from the Telfa to be analyzed by the pathologist.

7. The cervix is dried of any blood. Some physicians elect to spray the cervix for 3 to 5 seconds with topical 20% benzocaine spray. Excess fluid is wiped from below the cervix. This may provide pain relief during the biopsy procedure.

8. Biopsies are now to be performed, sampling the most abnormal-appearing areas. The number of biopsies is determined by the cervical appearance and the extent of diseased tissue. Performing fewer biopsies should not be encouraged, as each biopsy induces local immune response and can help in the resolution of cervical dysplasia. Biopsies on the posterior lip are performed first; bleeding from the initial biopsy will not interfere with subsequent biopsies on the anterior tip.

9. The biopsy instrument is positioned over the recorded abnormal-appearing site on the cervix. The fixed portion of the biopsy instrument should be within the canal, with the moveable portion of the biopsy instrument over the ectocervix (Figure 1.2). The tips of the instrument

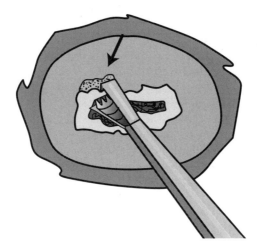

FIGURE 1.2. Once the most abnormal areas are identified by examination through the colposcope, biopsy is performed. The biopsy instrument is positioned so the fixed portion is within the canal, and the mobile portion is on the outside. Biopsy is performed at the 11 o'clock position.

TABLE 1.2.   CPT Codes

CPT Codes	Description	1998 Total RVUs[a]	1998 Average 50% Fees in U.S.[b]
57452	Colposcopy [vaginoscopy]; [separate procedure]	1.78	$200
57454	Colposcopy with Bx and/or ECC	2.74	$275
57460	Colposcopy with LEEP	5.31	$750
57500	Biopsy of the cervix only	1.66	$131
57505	ECC only	1.90	$141

CPT only © 1998 American Medical Association. All rights reserved.

[a]Department of Health and Human Services, Health Care Financing Administration. Medicare program: revisions to payment policies and adjustments to the relative value units (RVUs) under the physician fee schedule for calendar year 1998. Federal Register 42 CFR part 414. October 31, 1997; 62(211):59103–59255.

[b]1998 Physicians' Fee Reference. West Allis, WI: Yale Wasserman, DMD, Medical Publishers, 1998.

can be partially closed, and the tissue grasped before the biopsy is obtained. Firm, rapid pressure should be applied to the biopsy handle in order to obtain an adequate and appropriate-sized biopsy. If the instrument is pushed too far into the cervix, a very large bite of tissue can be obtained. Deep bites can be painful. If the instrument is not adequately applied to the tissue, only the surface of the cervix will be scraped, yielding an inadequate specimen.

10. Biopsies can be freed from the biopsy instruments using toothpicks. Due to the excessive costs generated by placing individual biopsies in individual containers, all the ectocervical biopsies are placed in one specimen container. The sites of the biopsies are marked on the procedure recording form.

11. As soon as the biopsies are completed, a dry, large, cotton-tipped swab is used to apply pressure to the cervix. A second swab can begin to remove the blood from below the cervix. Monsel's solution is applied to small or large cotton-tipped swabs. As the drying/pressure swab is removed from the cervix, the other hand applies the swab with the Monsel's solution on it. This process may need to be repeated several times. Monsel's solution is best applied to a dry wound bed. If a bloody wound bed is present, a thick brown coagulum is created. The coagulum may prevent the Monsel's solution from reaching the wound bed, affecting hemostasis. With experience, the physician can learn to apply the Monsel's solution quickly and effectively.

12. Once the cervix has achieved adequate hemostasis, any debris or brown coagulum in the posterior fornix is removed from below the cervix with a dry, large, cotton-tipped swab. The speculum is gently removed, and an absorbent pad is given to the patient to place in the underwear (Monsel's solution can stain the underwear). Allow the patient to get dressed before the final conference with the physician.

FOLLOW UP

See Table 1.3 for an explanation of colposcopy terminology.

* Disease inside the endocervical canal is felt by many to have greater prognostic significance. Whenever any squamous dysplasia, including mild dysplasia (cervical intraepithelial neoplasia [CIN] 1), is found in the endocervi-

TABLE 1.3. Colposcopy Terminology

NORMAL COLPOSCOPY FINDINGS
Original squamous epithelium
Columnar epithelium
Normal transformation zone, including Nabothian cysts and metaplasia

ABNORMAL COLPOSCOPY FINDINGS
Acetowhite epithelium
Leukoplakia (condyloma)
Vascular changes of punctation or mosaic
Atypical vessels
Inflammation (friable, exudate, discharge)
Atrophy
Surface contour changes (exophytic mass, ulceration)

UNSATISFACTORY COLPOSCOPY
Entire squamocolumnar junction not visible
Severe inflammation or severe atrophy
Cervix not visualized (cervix retracted to side, obese patient)

COLPOSCOPY CHANGES

Minor Changes—Suggesting Low-grade Dysplastic Changes
Acetowhite epithelium
Fine mosaic
Fine punctation
Thin leukoplakia

Major Changes—Suggesting High-grade Dysplastic or Cancerous Changes
Dense acetowhite epithelium
Coarse mosaic
Coarse punctation
Thick leukoplakia
Atypical vessels
Erosion

Adapted from Stafl A, Wilbanks GD. An international terminology of colposcopy: report of the nomenclature committee of the international federation of cervical pathology and colposcopy. Obstet Gynecol 1991; 77:313–314.

cal canal, many experts recommend a conization. Adenocarcinoma in situ in the canal should prompt referral or consideration for conization.

- The presence of high-grade dysplasia (CIN 2 or 3) of the cervix should prompt consideration of a surgical procedure. Some experts also recommend treatment if the colposcopic visual impression, histologic (biopsy) result, and cytologic (Pap) result do not agree within one grade. For example, surgical treatment can be considered if the Pap suggests CIN 3, even if the biopsies only demonstrate CIN 1 (a two-grade discrepancy). LEEP, laser excision or ablation, or cryosurgery can be considered for surgical intervention. Cryosurgery can have lower cure rates for CIN 3 that is present in multiple quadrants of the cervix. The choice of therapy should not be influenced by lack of physician performance of an appropriate therapy, such as LEEP.

- While there is no consensus on the best treatment for mild squamous dysplasia of the cervix, many experts now recognize the low malignant potential of CIN 1. Because of the high rates of spontaneous resolution of CIN 1, strategies for following this abnormality have been developed. Studies have demonstrated the safety and efficacy of following mild dysplasia for up to 3 years. Strategies for following mild dysplasia are not completely risk-free; patients need to be aware that 1% of even the lowest grade dysplasia can progress to cancer. If a patient chooses to follow up on the mild abnormality, Pap smears can be performed at 4 and 8 months following the colposcopy. If these Pap smears are completely normal, a third Pap smear should be done 12 months after the colposcopy. If it is normal, the patient is returned to routine annual follow up. If the follow-up Pap smears are abnormal, many experts recommend a follow-up colposcopy 1 year after the initial study to evaluate the status of the cervix.

- HPV changes are frequently discovered at colposcopy. One goal of therapy for HPV lesions is to induce an immune response to the HPV, allowing the body to keep the virus in check. Smokers should be encouraged to discontinue smoking, as smoking can significantly interfere with immune response to HPV and permit dysplasia to persist. Because immune function can be influenced by nutritional deficiencies, patients can be encouraged to take vitamins, and, possibly, an antioxidant.

- Schedule a follow-up visit 1 month after colposcopy. The cervix can be treated at that visit, if needed. If the patient chooses to follow up on low-grade changes, use the follow-up visit to ensure that the patient understands the importance of follow-up within the next year and the schedule for these visits.

- The presence of invasive cervical cancer in the cervical biopsies should prompt consideration of referral to a gynecologic oncologist. Other referrals may be appropriate, especially if a confusing or uncertain biopsy result is obtained.

PROCEDURE PITFALLS/COMPLICATIONS

- *An adequate biopsy specimen was not obtained.* Novice colposcopists often do not want to hurt the patient and they tend to make halfhearted attempts at biopsy. The result that is often obtained is a scraping of the cervical tissue. Once the local anesthetic has been administered, the biopsy forceps should be correctly positioned. The teeth of the instrument should gently grasp the tissue and a quick, but firm, bite of the tissue should be obtained.

- *The patient developed cancer, even though the colposcopic biopsies were normal.* Several studies have demonstrated that colposcopic biopsies can underestimate the extent of cervical disease. The physician can biopsy the wrong area or inadequate biopsy specimens can be obtained. Some cavalier colposcopists may forego the biopsies or ECC, but experienced colposcopists understand the need for biopsies to confirm their clinical impressions. The colposcopist must interpret the biopsy results in light of the clinical impression and cytology (Pap smear) results. Further investigation should be undertaken if histologic undercall is suspected.

- *The Pap smear suggested adenomatous atypia, but the cervical biopsies just revealed squamous dysplasia.* Because adenomatous atypia can progress to adenocarcinoma at a rapid rate, colposcopic evaluation is recommended. Interestingly, about 75% of patients with adenomatous atypia exhibit only squamous cell abnormalities on biopsy and ECC evaluation. If the source for adenomatous changes cannot be identified on the cervix, endometrial biopsy and vaginal examination through the colposcope is recommended.

- *The biopsy site continued bleeding for several minutes, despite the application of Monsel's solution.* Monsel's (ferric subsulfate) solution is a hemostatic agent that works best on a dry wound bed. Novice physicians may have difficulty drying blood from the biopsy site before the Monsel's solution is applied. The correct technique requires two hands: one hand uses a cotton-tipped applicator to dry the wound bed, and as the first swab is being removed, the other hand slips the Monsel's solution onto the wound bed. If the Monsel's solution is applied to a bloody field, a thick, brownish-black coagulum develops. This coagulum can prevent the Monsel's solution from reaching the vessels at the base of the wound, and bleeding can persist even though the brownish-black coagulum is present.

- *The patient experienced intensive cramping during the procedure.* Uterine cramping commonly develops during and after colposcopic examination. The endocervical curettage may cause extensive cramping. Efforts aimed to reduce patient discomfort, such as preprocedure ibuprofen and the use of sharp instruments, may help.

PHYSICIAN TRAINING

Physicians should use multiple learning modalities for the development of colposcopic skills. Intensive, 2- or 3-day colposcopy courses can provide the basic knowledge and skills needed to perform the procedure. Precepted procedures with skilled colposcopists should be performed prior to initiating unsupervised procedure. Most physicians feel comfortable with the basic procedure after five to 10 precepted cases. Colposcopic skills can be sharpened by studying videotapes, atlases, and slide sets.

COLPOSCOPY TEACHING RESOURCES

Books

Handbook of Colposcopy (paperback). K.D. Hatch. Little, Brown & Co., Boston, MA.

Practical Colposcopy (color colposcopy atlas). R. Cartier. Gustav Fischer Verlag, New York, NY (can be obtained from Cabot Medical, 800-523-6078).

Colposcopy Text and Atlas (black and white atlas). L. Burke. Appleton & Lange, Norwalk, CT.

Videotape

Colposcopy for the Primary Care Physician. J. Pfenninger. CME conference video, Mt. Laurel, NJ; 800-284-8433.

Slide Teaching Set with Videotape and Manual

Modern Colposcopy. M.J. Campion. Cabot Medical, Langhorne, PA 19047; 800-523-6078.

Slide Teaching Sets and Videotapes

Colposcopy Studies. D. Townsend. Physician Educational Network, Sacremento, CA; 916-454-5939.

HPV-Related Diseases. A. Ferenczy. BioVision, New York.

ORDERING INFORMATION

Formalin containers (CMS Protocol 10% neutral buffered formalin 30 mL, Biochemical Science, Swedesboro, NJ 08085; 800-524-0294)

Large Graves' vaginal speculum, Foerster (ring) forceps (straight, 9 ½ inches, serrated jaws), Tischler biopsy forceps (3 × 7 mm bite, 8 ¼-inch shaft), Kevorkian-Younge endocervical biopsy curette (12 inch, loop size 3 × 12 mm, without basket) (Miltex Instrument Co, 6 Ohio Drive, Lake Success, NY 11042; 800-645-8000)

Colposcope (Olympus Corporation, 3900 Kilroy Airport Way, Suite 100, Long Beach, CA 90806; 800-626-1917)

BIBLIOGRAPHY

ACOG Technical Bulletin #183. Cervical cytology: evaluation and management of abnormalities. Washington, DC: American College of Obstetrics and Gynecology, 1993:1–8.

American Academy of Family Physicians. Basic colposcopy for the family physician. Kansas City, MO: AAFP, 1992.

Burke L, Antonioli DA, Ducatman BS. Colposcopy text and atlas. Norwalk, CT: Appleton & Lange, 1991.

Cartier R. Practical colposcopy. Stuttgart: Gustav Fischer Verlag, 1984.

Centers for Disease Control. Human papillomavirus infection. MMWR 1993;42:83–88.

Hatch KD. Handbook of colposcopy: diagnosis and treatment of lower genital tract neoplasia and HPV infections. Boston: Little, Brown, 1989.

Hopman EH, Voorhorst FJ, Kenemans P, Meyer CJ, Helmerhorst TJ. Observer agreement on interpreting colposcopic images of CIN. Gynecol Oncol 1995;58:206–209.

Richart RM, Wright TC. Controversies in the management of low-grade cervical intraepithelial neoplasia. Cancer 1993;71:1413–1421.

Schiffman MH, Bauer HM, Hoover RN, et al. Epidemiologic evidence showing that human papillomavirus infection causes most cervical intraepithelial neoplasia. J Natl Cancer Inst 1993;85:958–964.

Skehan M, Soutter WP, Lim K, Krausz T, Pryse-Davies J. Reliability of colposcopy and directed punch biopsy. Br J Obstet Gynecol 1990;97:811–816.

Zuber TJ. The minimally abnormal Pap smear: a conservative approach (Editorial). Am Fam Physician 1996;53:1042,1048,1050.

CHAPTER 2

Endometrial Biopsy

Endometrial biopsy is a safe and accepted method for the evaluation of abnormal or postmenopausal bleeding. The procedure is often performed to exclude the presence of endometrial cancer or its precursors (Tables 2.1 and 2.2). The office endometrial suction catheters are easy to use, and several have been reported to have diagnostic accuracy that is equal or superior to the dilatation and curettage (D&C) procedure. Suction is generated by withdrawing an internal piston from within the catheter, and the tissue sample is obtained by twirling the catheter, while moving it up and down within the uterine cavity.

Endometrial biopsy is a blind procedure, and should be considered part of the evaluation that could include imaging studies, such as hysteroscopy or transvaginal ultrasonography. While a negative study is reassuring, further evaluation is warranted if a patient demonstrates continued abnormal bleeding.

METHODS AND MATERIALS

Equipment

Nonsterile Tray for Examination for Uterine Position

  Nonsterile gloves

  Lubricating jelly

  Absorbent pad to place beneath the patient on the examination table

  Formalin container (for endometrial sample) with the patient's name and the date recorded on the label

  20% Benzocaine (Hurricaine) spray with the extended application nozzle

Sterile Tray for the Procedure

Place the following items on a sterile drape covering the Mayo stand with the following items placed on top:

  Sterile gloves

  Sterile vaginal speculum

  Uterine sound

TABLE 2.1.   Indications for Endometrial Biopsy

Abnormal uterine bleeding
Postmenopausal bleeding
Cancer screening (e.g., hereditary nonpolyposis colorectal cancer)
Detection of precancerous hyperplasia and atypia
Endometrial dating
Follow up of previously diagnosed endometrial hyperplasia
Evaluation of uterine response to hormone therapy
Evaluation of patient with 1 year of amenorrhea
Evaluation of infertility
Abnormal Pap smear with atypical cells favoring endometrial origin

> Sterile metal basin containing sterile cotton balls soaked in povidone-iodine solution
>
> Endometrial suction catheter
>
> Cervical tenaculum
>
> Ring forceps (for wiping the cervix with the cotton balls)
>
> Sterile 4 × 4 gauze (to wipe off gloves or equipment)
>
> Sterile scissors (if the physician chooses to cut off the catheter tip to deliver the endometrial sample into the formalin container).

Keep sterile cervical dilators available, but do not open the sterile packaging unless the dilators are needed.

Once the physician is sterile gloved and has placed the speculum, the nurse can spray the benzocaine spray onto the cervix for 5 seconds, avoiding contamination of the sterile speculum with the extended spray nozzle.

TABLE 2.2.   Contraindications and Relative Contraindications
for Endometrial Biopsy

CONTRAINDICATIONS
Pregnancy
Acute pelvic inflammatory disease (PID)
Clotting disorders (coagulopathy)
Acute cervical or vaginal infections
Cervical cancer

CONDITIONS POSSIBLY PROHIBITING ENDOMETRIAL BIOPSY
Morbid obesity
Severe pelvic relaxation with uterine descensus
Severe cervical stenosis

PROCEDURE DESCRIPTION

1. The patient is placed in the lithotomy position and bimanual examination is performed (with nonsterile gloves) to determine the uterine size and position, and whether marked uterocervical angulation exists. Still wearing the nonsterile gloves, the physician can pick up the sterile speculum from the sterile tray and place it in the patient's vagina. Avoid contaminating the sterile instruments on the tray. Once the cervix is centered in the speculum, the cervix can be anesthetized by spraying 20% benzocaine spray for 5 seconds, and then cleansing it with povidone-iodine solution.

2. Alternately, the physician can apply sterile gloves, and insert the sterile speculum into the patient's vagina. The physician should minimize contact of the sterile gloves with the nonsterile vulvar tissues. The cervix is centered in the speculum and cleansed with povidone-iodine solution. The gloves can be washed with povidone-iodine solution if contaminated. The nurse can then spray the cervix with the 20% benzocaine spray for 5 seconds, avoiding contamination of the sterile speculum with the extended spray nozzle.

3. The cervix is gently probed with the uterine sound. The cervix often is too mobile to allow for passage of the sound, but can be stabilized with the tenaculum. The tenaculum is placed on the anterior lip of the cervix, grabbing enough tissue that the cervix will not lacerate when traction is applied. The author prefers placement of the tenaculum in most cases, for increased safety, and grasps the anterior lip of the cervix with the tenaculum teeth in the horizontal plane.

4. Pull outward on the tenaculum gently, straightening the uterocervical angle to reduce the chance of posterior perforation. Attempt to insert the uterine sound to the fundus. Occasionally, steady, moderate pressure is required to insert the sound through the closed internal cervical os.

5. If the uterine sound will not pass through the internal os, consider placement of small Pratt uterine dilators. The smallest size is inserted, followed by insertion of successively larger dilators until the sound passes easily to the fundus. The distance from the fundus to the external cervical os can be measured by the gradations on the uterine sound, and generally will be 6 to 8 cm.

6. The endometrial biopsy catheter tip is inserted into the cervix, avoiding contamination from the nearby tissues. The catheter tip is then inserted into the uterine fundus, or until resistance is felt (Fig. 2.1A). Once the catheter is in the uterine cavity, the internal piston on the catheter is fully withdrawn (Fig. 2.1B), creating suction at the catheter tip. The catheter tip is moved with an in-and-out motion, but the tip does not exit the endometrial cavity through the cervix, which maintains the vacuum effect. Use a 360° twisting motion to move the catheter between the

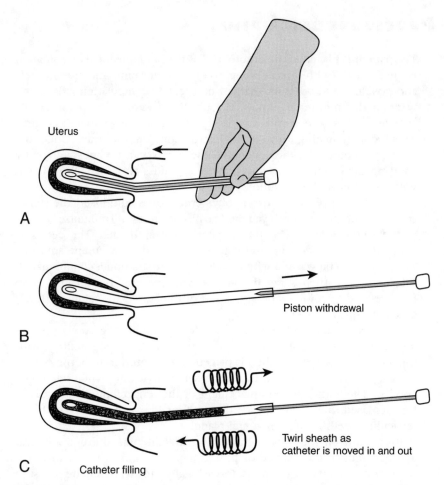

Uterus

A

Piston withdrawal

B

Twirl sheath as
catheter is moved in and out

C   Catheter filling

FIGURE 2.1. **A.** The catheter tip is inserted into the uterus fundus or until resistance is felt. **B.** Once the catheter is in the uterus cavity, the internal piston is fully withdrawn. **C.** Use a 360° twisting motion as the catheter is moved between the uterus fundus and the internal os.

uterine fundus and the internal cervical os (Fig. 2.1C). Make at least four up and down excursions to ensure that adequate tissue is in the catheter.

7. Once the catheter fills with tissue, it is withdrawn and the sample is placed in the formalin container. To remove the sample from the endometrial catheter, the piston can be gently reinserted, forcing the tissue out of the catheter tip. Some physicians prefer to make a second pass into the uterus with the catheter to optimize tissue sampling. If a second pass is to be made, the catheter should not be contaminated when being emptied of the first specimen.

TABLE 2.3.   CPT Codes for Endoscopy

CPT Codes	Description	1998 Total RVUs[a]	1998 Average 50% Fees in U.S.[b]
58100	Endometrial biopsy—no dilation	1.51	$161
57800	Cervical dilation—instrumental [separate procedure]	1.35	$150
59200	Cervical dilation—laminaria, prostaglandin [separate procedure]	1.44	$153

CPT only © 1998 American Medical Association. All rights reserved.
[a]Department of Health and Human Services, Health Care Financing Administration. Medicare program: revisions to payment policies and adjustments to the relative value units (RVUs) under the physician fee schedule for calendar year 1998. Federal Register 42 CFR part 414. October 31, 1997; 62(211):59103–59255.
[b]1998 Physicians' Fee Reference. West Allis, WI: Yale Wasserman, DMD, Medical Publishers, 1998.

8. The tenaculum is gently removed. Pressure can be applied with cotton swabs if the tenaculum sites bleed following removal of the tenaculum. Excess blood and povidone-iodine solution are wiped from the vagina, and the vaginal speculum is removed.

FOLLOW UP

- Normal endometrial tissue may be described as proliferative (estrogen effect or preovulatory) endometrium or secretory (progesterone effect or postovulatory) endometrium. Hormone therapy can be offered to patients with abnormal vaginal bleeding who have normal endometrial tissue on biopsy. If the biopsy is normal but the patient continues to experience excessive vaginal bleeding, further diagnostic workup should occur.
- Atrophic endometrium generally yields scant or insufficient tissue for diagnosis. Hormonal therapy may be considered for patients with atrophic endometrium. Persistent vaginal bleeding should warrant further diagnostic workup.
- Cystic or simple hyperplasia progresses to cancer in less than 5% of patients. Most individuals with simple hyperplasia without any atypia can be managed with hormonal manipulation (medroxyprogesterone [Provera], 10 mg daily for 5 days to 3 months) or with close follow up. Most authors recommend a follow-up endometrial biopsy after 3 to 12 months, regardless of the management strategy.
- Atypical complex hyperplasia is a premalignant lesion that progresses to cancer in 30 to 45% of women. Some physicians will treat complex hyperplasia with or without atypia with hormonal therapy (medroxyprogesterone, 10 to 20 mg daily for up to 3 months). Most physicians recommend a D&C procedure to exclude the presence of endometrial carcinoma, and consider hysterectomy for complex or high-grade hyperplasia.

• Biopsy specimens that suggest the presence of endometrial carcinoma (75% are adenocarcinoma) should prompt consideration of referral to a gynecologic oncologist for definitive surgical therapy.

PROCEDURE PITFALLS/COMPLICATIONS

• *The catheter won't go up into the uterus easily in perimenopausal patients.* The internal cervical os may be very tight in perimenopausal and menopausal patients. Because of the discomfort that can be created by instrumental cervical dilation, an alternative in older patients is to insert an osmotic laminaria (seaweed) 3 mm dilator in the patient that morning. Osmotic dilators cause gentle, slow opening of the cervix. The osmotic dilator is removed in the afternoon, and then the endometrial biopsy can easily be performed.

• *Patients report cramping associated with the procedure.* Intraoperative and postoperative cramping frequently accompany instrumentation of the uterine cavity. Preprocedure oral nonsteroidal anti-inflammatory medications, such as ibuprofen (Motrin), can significantly reduce the prostaglandin-induced cramping. Spraying the cervix with a topical anesthetic, such as 20% benzocaine, can also help with discomfort.

• *The procedure should not be performed in pregnant patients.* Endometrial biopsy should not be performed in the presence of a normal or ectopic pregnancy. All patients with the potential for pregnancy should be considered for pregnancy testing prior to the performance of the procedure.

• *Infection occurs following the procedure.* Bacteremia, sepsis, and acute bacterial endocarditis have been reported following endometrial biopsy. Because postprocedure bacteremia has been noted, some authors recommend considering antibiotics in postmenopausal women at risk for endocarditis. The risk for infection appears to be small, but some physicians recommend tetracycline, 500 mg twice daily, for 4 days following the procedure.

• *The pathologist reports that the specimens have insufficient sample for diagnosis.* Some physicians are less vigorous in obtaining specimens, and a single pass of the catheter may not yield adequate tissue. A second pass can be made with the suction catheter if it is not contaminated when it is emptied after the first pass. The second pass almost always prevents reporting an insufficient sample.

• *The tenaculum causes discomfort when applied to the cervix.* Topical anesthesia can reduce the discomfort from the tenaculum. Placement of the tenaculum can make the procedure safer for the patient. The tenaculum stabilizes the cervix and allows the physician to straighten the uterocervical angle. The tenaculum can reduce the chances of posterior perforation when the plastic catheter is inserted through the cervix and then through the thin-walled lower uterine segment.

PHYSICIAN TRAINING

Endometrial biopsy is a fairly easy technique to learn. Physicians are often comfortable performing the procedure unassisted after two to five precepted procedures. Physicians who perform other gynecologic procedures find that endometrial biopsy is a natural addition to their practices. The American Academy of Family Physicians offers a comprehensive training course in endometrial biopsy for physicians wanting intensive training.

ORDERING INFORMATION

Formalin containers CMS Protocol (10% neutral buffered formalin, 30 cc, Biochemical Science, 200 Commodore Drive, Swedesboro, NJ 08085; 800-524-0294)

Hurricane 20% topical anesthetic spray (60 g bottle, Beutlich Inc, 1541 Shields Drive, Waukegan, IL 60085; 847-473-1100)

Unimar Pipelle endometrial suction catheter (Cooper Surgical, 15 Forest Parkway, Shelton, CT 06484; 800-243-6608)

Graves medium vaginal speculum, Pratt uterine 7½ inch double-end dilators (13-15 Fr., 17-19 Fr., 21-23 Fr., 25-27 Fr.), Simpson uterine sound 13 inch malleable, Foerster sponge (ring) forceps 9½ inch straight with serrated jaws, Schroeder-Braun uterine tenaculum forceps 9¾ inch straight (Miltex Instrument Co, 6 Ohio Drive, Lake Success, NY 11042; 800-645-8000)

Osmotic dilators (Lamicel, Circon Surgitek, 3037 Mount Pleasant Street, Racine, WI 53404; 800-523-6078)

BIBLIOGRAPHY

Baughan DM. Office endometrial aspiration biopsy. Fam Pract Res 1993;15:45-55.

Bayer SR, DeCherney AH. Clinical manifestations and treatment of dysfunctional uterine bleeding. JAMA 1993;269:1823-1828.

Bremer CC. Endometrial biopsy. Female Patient 1992;17:15-28.

Grimes DA. Diagnostic dilation and curettage: a reappraisal. Am J Obstet Gynecol 1982;142:1-6.

Kaunitz AM. Endometrial sampling in menopausal patients. Menopausal Med 1993;1:5-8.

Kaunitz AM, Masciello A, Ostrowski M, Rovira EZ. Comparison of endometrial biopsy with the endometrial Pipelle and Vabra aspirator. J Reprod Med 1988;33:427-431.

Livengood CH, Land MR, Addison A. Endometrial biopsy, bacteremia, and endocarditis risk. Obstet Gynecol 1985;65:678–681.

Mettlin C, Jones G, Averette H, Gusberg SB, Murphy GP. Defining and updating the American Cancer Society Guidelines for the cancer-related check-up: prostate and endometrial cancers. CA Cancer J Clin 1993;43:42–46.

Nesse RE. Managing abnormal vaginal bleeding. Postgrad Med 1991;89:205–208, 213–214.

Reagan MA, Isaacs JH. Office diagnosis of endometrial carcinoma. Prim Care Cancer 1992;12:49–52.

Esophagogastroduodenoscopy

Esophagogastroduodenoscopy (EGD) provides the physician with an excellent view of the mucosal surfaces of the upper gastrointestinal tract. EGD has been demonstrated to be diagnostically superior to gastrointestinal radiographic studies. The procedure is advocated in the evaluation of many abdominal and chest complaints.

The office setting can be advantageous to both patient and physician, and is increasingly chosen for the performance of EGD. It has been suggested that primary care endoscopy procedures improve health care quality, patient access to care, cost factors, physicians' relationships with patients, and physicians' understanding of the involved pathology. Alternative, nonintravenous methods of sedation and pain control have been demonstrated to support complete and well-tolerated procedures in the office setting. Good patient outcomes often follow proper patient selection, avoidance of medically unstable patients, and referral of therapeutic or high-risk procedures to a more carefully monitored setting (such as the hospital).

For non-intravenous sedation, it has been recommended that patients take 0.25 or 0.5 mg of oral triazolam (Halcion) 1 hour before the procedure. Butorphanol tartrate nasal spray (Stadol) can be administered immediately prior to the procedure, if additional sedation is desired. Topical anesthesia with 2% lidocaine jelly (Xylocaine) and 20% benzocaine spray (Hurricane) enhance the patient's comfort. A pediatric (7.9 to 9.0 mm diameter) endoscope can be used for additional comfort and safety. Patients should be monitored by continuous cardiac monitor, oximetry, and blood pressure recordings. This protocol avoids patient discomfort, cost, and risk of intravenous lines and medication administration. Patient acceptance of this protocol has been high.

A major advantage of endoscopy over radiographic study is the ability to perform biopsies. The performance of biopsies is an important component of EGD, and accurate placement of the biopsy tip can determine the correct histologic evaluation of small polyps or large gastric ulcers. Biopsy is also performed to determine the presence of *Helicobacter pylori*. *H. pylori* can be detected by histology or by the performance of urease testing (CLOtest). *H. pylori* produces a large amount of urease, which hydrolyzes urea to ammonia. The CLOtest produces a color change from the resulting ammonia.

23

Most EGD procedures performed by family physicians result in a change in the patient's diagnosis or management. Due to the cost and invasive nature of the procedure, many experts recommend that the procedure be performed in the evaluation of patients with symptoms of acid-peptic disorders only after a trial of medication therapy. Patients with signs of serious organic disease (e.g., anorexia or weight loss), or who have upper abdominal distress may benefit from more prompt evaluation. The indications and contraindications are listed in Tables 3.1 and 3.2.

METHODS AND MATERIALS

Patient Preparation

The patient is placed in the left lateral decubitus position, with the head flexed and supported on a pillow, and knees slightly bent. The arms are placed at the patient's side. Absorbent pads are placed beneath the patient's head and neck. Oximeter and cardiac monitors are placed.

Equipment

Nonsterile Tray

Place the following items on a nonsterile sheet covering the Mayo stand:

Nonsterile gloves and mask

1 inch of 4 × 4 gauze

Butorphanol spray

Medicine cup filled with 10 mL viscous 2% lidocaine and fruit flavoring

TABLE 3.1.   Some of the Indications for Diagnostic EGD

Dyspepsia unresponsive to medical therapy
Persistent dysphagia or odynophagia
Persistent vomiting of unknown cause
Evaluation of an abnormal radiographic finding
Esophageal reflux symptoms that are persistent or unresponsive to therapy
Evaluation of upper gastrointestinal bleeding
Upper abdominal distress associated with serious signs such as weight loss
Iron deficiency anemia following negative colon evaluation
Chest pain with negative cardiac workup
Periodic surveillance of proven Barrett's esophagus
Follow up of selected gastric ulcers to document clearance
Familial polyposis or Gardner's syndrome
Follow up of previously diagnosed adenomatous gastric polyps
Suspected malabsorption (for small bowel biopsy)
Persistent regurgitation of undigested food

TABLE 3.2. Some of the Contraindications to Office EGD

Known or suspected perforated viscus
Acute, severe, or unstable cardiopulmonary disease
Uncooperative patient
Severe or active upper gastrointestinal bleeding
Patient who may require therapeutic EGD
Valvular heart disease without antibiotic prophylaxis
Hemodynamically unstable patient

A disposable plastic spoon for administering the viscous lidocaine

20% benzocaine spray

2 CLOtest testing wells

1 inch of 2% lidocaine jelly on 4×4 gauze (for scope lubrication)

Mouth guard

Endoscopy Cart

EGD scope connected to a light source, camera, and video screen

Suction and water channels connected and tested for proper functioning

Biopsy forceps

Oximetry monitor

Cardiac monitor with leads

Automated blood pressure recording unit

PROCEDURE DESCRIPTION

1. The patient is placed in the left lateral decubitus position, with the head flexed and supported on a pillow, and knees slightly bent. The arms are placed at the patient's side. Absorbent pads are placed beneath the patient's head and neck. Oximeter and cardiac monitors are placed. The nurse completes the preprocedure nursing checklist.
2. The patient is given 1 teaspoon of 2% lidocaine viscous solution mixed with 2 drops of fruit flavoring. The patient gargles the solution in the throat, and then swallows the solution. Another teaspoon of this solution is administered just before starting the procedure, after the administration of benzocaine spray. One or two sprays of butorphanol can be administered intranasally if the patient is anxious or if additional sedation is desired.
3. The patient's throat is sprayed with 20% benzocaine spray. The patient should hold his or her breath during the spraying to keep from pulling the spray into the nasal cavity. The spray has an unpleasant taste, and

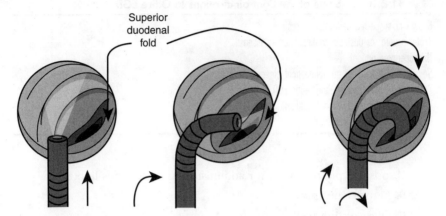

FIGURE 3.1. In 70% of patients, the path into the descending duodenum is not a straight shot. The scope may need to be torqued clockwise while turning the top to the right in order to slip around the superior duodenal fold and loop into the descending duodenum.

the patient may cough or gag following administration. The patient's mouth is covered with gauze immediately after the spraying to limit fluid expulsion during coughing. The examiner's finger can confirm anesthesia to the posterior tongue. The second teaspoon of viscous lidocaine is given as a chaser, to reduce the flavor of the benzocaine.

4. The patient's neck is flexed, and the chin is brought down near the upper chest. The mouth guard is carefully inserted between the upper and lower front teeth, and the patient should be instructed to maintain enough pressure to prevent the mouth guard from moving during the procedure.

5. The distal portion of the endoscope is then lubricated with 2% lidocaine jelly. The scope tip is inserted through the mouth guard, and flexed over the back of the tongue and positioned to where the structures of the larynx can be visualized. The jelly is kept off the most distal tip to avoid smearing the lens and distorting the image. The scope tip is positioned just posterior to the vocal cords, above the cricopharyngeus muscle. Avoid touching the walls of the hypopharynx or larynx, which will cause gagging.

6. Entry into the esophagus is performed by the direct vision technique. Once the scope tip is positioned, ask the patient to swallow. As the swallowing motion starts, the cricopharyngeus opens and the scope is gently advanced until the lumen of the upper esophagus appears. This is the most difficult part of the procedure for the patient, because

coughing and gagging may occur. Several attempts may be needed for esophageal intubation. Proper positioning of the scope tip, and rapid-but-gentle tip advancement can facilitate intubation.

7. The esophagus is viewed as the scope passes through to the stomach. The cricopharyngeus is located at about the 18 cm insertion point, and the esophagus is about 20 cm long. The pale, pink esophageal mucosa terminates at the Z-line, and the deep orange-red gastric mucosa can be seen beyond. The area is inspected for a hiatal hernia or pathology. The diaphragmatic indentation should be noted by having the diaphragm contract (i.e., have the patient sniff). A hiatal hernia exists when the Z-line is more than 2 cm above the diaphragmatic indentation (Fig. 3.1).

8. The scope enters the stomach, and air is insufflated to expand the lumen. The scope tip is turned into the gastric lake, and the secretions and anesthetic solutions are suctioned out to reduce the chance of aspiration.

9. The stomach is rapidly traversed, and the pyloric opening is viewed. Pylorospasm may develop from the presence of the scope in the stomach, and some experts advise duodenal intubation before extensive examination of the stomach. Persistence may be needed to intubate the duodenum. The scope tip is positioned just outside the pylorus, air is applied, and the scope is inserted as the pylorus opens with peristalsis.

10. The scope should be brought into the descending duodenum. Thirty percent of patients have a straight passage into the second portion of the duodenum, but 70% require torquing (to the right) around the superior duodenal angle (Fig. 3.1).

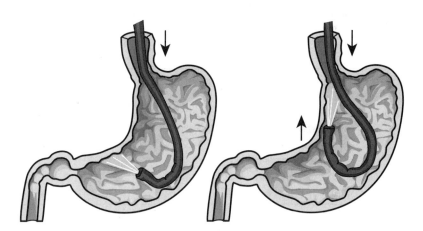

FIGURE 3.2. The endoscope is retroverted to examine the fundus and gastroesophageal junction from below. This maneuver is recommended because the incidence of carcinoma at this location is increasing.

11. The duodenum and all four walls of the duodenal bulb must be examined. Often the scope tip slips back into the stomach, and the pylorus must be reintubated to reexamine the duodenal bulb. Once the duodenum is examined, the scope is withdrawn into the stomach.

12. The gastric mucosa is thoroughly examined. The scope tip is curved to view the sharp incisura or angularis of the lesser curvature of the stomach. With the scope tip completely curled, the scope can be withdrawn to allow for viewing the scope entering the stomach. This retroflexion maneuver allows for inspection of the cardia and fundus of the stomach (Fig. 3.1). Another sniff test can be performed to examine the diaphragmatic indentations from below, and to look for a hiatal hernia.

13. The scope is straightened and two antral biopsies are performed for CLOtesting. Additional biopsies or brushings may be performed to evaluate any pathology or areas that appear abnormal.

14. The scope is withdrawn to the upper stomach and the air in the stomach is removed. The scope is withdrawn into the distal esophagus, and this area reexamined. The esophagus is examined as the scope is withdrawn.

15. After removal of the scope and mouth guard, secretions that have drained onto the patient's cheek are wiped with gauze. The patient is placed on his or her back, and the nurse completes the postprocedure nursing checklist.

16. After completing the paperwork and giving the patient a brief rest, the postprocedure conference can be held to review the study findings. It is often best to include any family members who may be present because the sedative medications can cause the patient to forget the issues discussed.

TABLE 3.3. CPT Codes for EGD

CPT Codes	Description	1998 Total RVUs[a]	1998 Average 50% Fees in U.S.[b]
43234	Upper EGD, simple primary examination [separate procedure]	4.88	$473
43235	Upper EGD, diagnostic, with or without collection of specimen(s) by brushing or washing [separate procedure]	5.75	$550
43239	EGD with biopsy, single or multiple	6.46	$608
94761	Oximetry, multiple readings	0.70	$54
99070	Surgical tray [A4550 for Medicare]	00	$32

CPT only © 1998 American Medical Association. All rights reserved.

[a]Department of Health and Human Services, Health Care Financing Administration. Medicare program: revisions to payment policies and adjustments to the relative value units (RVUs) under the physician fee schedule for calendar year 1998. Federal Register 42 CFR part 414. October 31, 1997;62(211):59103–59255.

[b]1998 Physicians' Fee Reference. West Allis, WI: Yale Wasserman, DMD, Medical Publishers, 1998.

FOLLOW UP

- Non-ulcer dyspepsia is a common finding in primary care practices. Patients may bitterly complain of symptoms, only to have normal findings at endoscopy. H_2 blockers and anxiolytics have been tried for this condition, with variable success.
- Patients with peptic ulcer disease who are positive for *H. pylori* (histology or CLOtest) should receive treatment. So-called triple drug therapy has been demonstrated to be moderately successful in eradicating *H. pylori*. Some controversy exists as to whether to treat individuals without endoscopic findings who are CLOtest positive. The presence of the bacteria appears to increase with age, and is found in many normal individuals, so many experts do not recommend treatment with normal endoscopic findings.
- Malignancy is commonly associated with gastric ulcers. Multiple biopsies should be taken when a gastric ulcer is found. If no malignant cells are noted, aggressive medical treatment can be initiated. Patients with a gastric ulcer should be reexamined in 2 to 4 months, and additional biopsies or consultation obtained if persisting ulceration is noted.
- Duodenal ulcers do not require repeat EGD examination, if the patient has responded adequately to treatment. Duodenal ulcers are highly associated with *H. pylori* infection, and the presence of the infection should be aggressively sought and treatment initiated.
- The presence of metaplastic gastric tissue in the esophagus, or Barrett's esophagus, should be sought in patients with long-standing reflux. Barrett's can be associated with dysplasia and subsequent cancer, and the presence of Barrett's requires periodic examination.
- When a gastric polyp is noted to be adenomatous, follow-up surveillance and biopsy are indicated.
- Certain findings may require therapeutic endoscopy, such as esophageal varices or peptic stricture. The presence of malignancy requires prompt referral. If the examiner discovers unusual or unfamiliar pathology, referral can be considered.

PROCEDURE PITFALLS/COMPLICATIONS

- *The patient coughs and gags when esophageal intubation is attempted.* Intubation of the esophagus is often the most difficult part of the procedure for both physician and patient. If the direct vision technique is used, the tip of the endoscope must be brought to just above the cricopharyngeus muscle. It is easy to touch the scope into side walls, thereby inducing a cough from the patient. Patients who are sleepy may require strong encouragement to swallow, thereby opening the cricopharyngeus and allowing intubation. Several attempts may be needed before the scope tip can be gently guided into the esophagus.

- *The patient developed aspiration pneumonia from the procedure.*
  Aspiration can occur during the intubation process, but it may be more
  likely to occur later in the procedure when the endoscope maintains
  mechanical opening of the upper and lower esophageal sphincters. To
  limit the likelihood or consequences of aspiration, it is recommended that
  the gastric lake be immediately suctioned once the stomach is intubated.

- *The patient developed a perforation following biopsy of a duodenal
  ulcer.* Unlike gastric ulcers, which must have a biopsy performed to exclude cancer, most duodenal ulcers do not require a biopsy. The term
  "ulcer" denotes the loss of tissue substance, and biopsy in the thin-walled
  duodenal bulb at a site with pathologic tissue loss can result in perforation.
  Biopsy should be undertaken for duodenal ulcers only when the appearance suggests an unusual or atypical finding or an associated mass lesion.

- *Oxygen saturation in an elderly patient drops during the procedure.* The most serious complications associated with EGD are cardiorespi-
  ratory events. Most cardiac arrhythmias or problems are preceded or associated with hypoxemia. Because oximetry monitoring is maintained during
  EGD, patients that develop hypoxemia receive supplemental oxygen. If
  the hypoxemia is severe or persistent, the procedure should be terminated.
  Larger endoscopes are associated with hypoxemia; use the smaller pediatric
  scopes. Excessive bowing of the gastric greater curvature by the scope,
  excessive insufflation of air into the stomach, or lengthy procedures may
  all be associated with hypoxemia.

- *Biopsy of the soft lesion produced excessive and prolonged bleeding.* Varices and angiomatous lesions should not have a biopsy done during
  diagnostic EGD. Beginning endoscopists are encouraged first to touch the
  lesions with the closed biopsy forceps tips to determine if the lesion is
  solid or compressible. If the lesion is compressible or soft, performing a
  biopsy should be deferred. Pulsating lesions should not be biopsied. Bleeding from biopsy sites in the stomach usually stops rapidly, due to the
  coagulating effects of the gastric acid. Excessive or pulsatile bleeding following a biopsy may require consultation, hospitalization, or therapeutic
  endoscopy.

- *The biopsy results returned nondiagnostic.* Nondiagnostic biopsy results are commonly seen by the beginning endoscopist, who is more likely
  to perform a biopsy on visually altered mucosa. A biopsy of gastric erythema
  often fails to yield useful information. Gastritis is a histologic diagnosis
  indicating inflammation, but the term often is misused to refer to gastric
  erythema. Large lesions that protrude into the lumen of the esophagus
  or stomach may also yield nondiagnostic biopsy results if the lesion is
  submucosal and the biopsy only samples the mucosal tissue. Smaller lesions
  can yield nondiagnostic biopsy results if the endoscopist fails to sample

directly over the abnormality. Beginning endoscopists must be precise in the selection of biopsy sites.

• ***The patient indicates discomfort or distress during the examination.*** Biopsy rarely causes significant discomfort during the procedure. If the patient indicates distress, usually an excessive amount of air has been placed in the stomach. Suctioning out the air can relieve the discomfort and allow the physician to resume the procedure. Efforts should be made to expedite the completion of the procedure, because patient tolerance decreases with longer procedures.

• ***The scope tip fails to advance through the pylorus despite insertion of the scope.*** It is easy to bow out the greater curvature of the stomach with insertion of the pediatric scope. Torquing the scope (twisting motion produced with the right hand on the scope) can effectively strengthen the scope tip and assist with insertion into the duodenal bulb. Once the duodenum has been intubated, withdrawal of the scope can actually produce a forward motion on the scope tip. The removal of the gastric bowing causes the paradoxical insertion.

PHYSICIAN TRAINING

Because of the complexity of the EGD procedure, and the multiple manual skills that must be mastered, formal training in this procedure is recommended. It is recommended that all physicians have at least 10 to 20 precepted examinations before attempting unsupervised EGDs. Many residency programs now provide training in diagnostic EGD. Formal courses in EGD, such as those offered by the American Academy of Family Physicians, can introduce the physician to the scope, anatomy, indications, complications, anesthesia, technique, and pathology of the upper gastrointestinal tract. Insertion of the scope into training models can aid in acquiring some of the manual skills. Study from textbooks, videotapes, and atlases can be beneficial. For the physician who wants to start performing EGD, prior experience in other endoscopic techniques (flexible sigmoidoscopy, colonoscopy) can facilitate the training.

ORDERING INFORMATION

Benzocaine 20% spray (Hurricaine, Beutlich Pharmaceuticals, 1541 Shields Drive, Waukegan, IL 60085; 800-238-8542)

Butorphanol tartrate spray (Stadol NS, Bristol-Myers Squibb Company, P.O. Box 4500, Princeton, NJ 08543; 800-332-2050)

CLOtest testing wells (Delta West Proprietary Ltd, Bently, Western Australia; Distributed by Tri-Med Specialties Inc, 16309 West 108th Circle, Lenexa, KS 66219; 913-888-4440)

Flexible EGD (7.9 mm or 9.0 mm diameter pediatric diagnostic) scope, mouth guard, biopsy forceps, light source, videoendoscopy screen (Olympus Corporation, 3900 Kilroy Airport Way, Suite 100, Long Beach, CA 90806; 800-626-1917)

Lidocaine jelly and viscous lidocaine (Xylocaine jelly and Xylocaine viscous, Astra U.S.A. Inc, Westborough, MA 01581, 508-366-1100, or through a local pharmacy)

Watermelon food flavoring (Lorann Oils, PO Box 22009, Lansing, MI 48909; 517-882-0215)

BIBLIOGRAPHY

The American Academy of Family Physicians. Esophagogastroduodenoscopy: a short course in basic skills and cognitive knowledge. Kansas City: AAFP, 1992.

American Society for Gastrointestinal Endoscopy. Appropriate use of gastrointestinal endoscopy: a consensus statement from the American Society for Gastrointestinal Endoscopy. Manchester, MA: ASGE, 1989.

Bytzer P, Hansen JM, Schaffalitzky de Muckadell OB. Empirical H_2-blocker therapy or prompt endoscopy in management of dyspepsia. Lancet 1994;343(8901):811–816.

Coleman WH. Gastroscopy: a primary diagnostic procedure. Prim Care 1988; 15:1–11.

Fleischer D. Monitoring the patient receiving conscious sedation for gastrointestinal endoscopy: issues and guidelines. Gastrointest Endosc 1989;35:262–266.

Health and Public Policy Committee, American College of Physicians. Clinical competence in diagnostic esophagogastroduodenoscopy. Ann Intern Med 1987; 107:937–939.

Health and Public Policy Committee, American College of Physicians. Endoscopy in the evaluation of dyspepsia. Ann Intern Med 1985;102:266–269.

Hocutt JE, Rodney WM, Zurad EG, Tucker RS, Norris T. Esophagogastroduodenoscopy for the family physician. Am Fam Physician 1994;49:109–116,121–122.

Rodney WM, Weber JR, Swedberg JA, et al. Esophagogastroduodenoscopy by family physicians phase II: a national multisite study of 2500 procedures. Fam Pract Res J 1993;13:121–131.

Woodliff DM. The role of upper gastrointestinal endoscopy in primary care. J Fam Pract 1979;8:715–719.

Zuber TJ. A pilot project in office-based diagnostic esophagogastroduodenoscopy comparing two nonintravenous methods of sedation and anesthesia. Arch Fam Med 1995;4:601–607.

RECOMMENDED ATLASES

Blackstone MO. Endoscopic interpretation: normal and pathologic appearances of the gastrointestinal tract. New York: Raven Press, 1984.

Schiller KF, Cockel R, Hunt RH, Ashby BS, Stevenson GW. A colour atlas of gastrointestinal endoscopy. Philadelphia: WB Saunders, 1986.

CHAPTER 4

Flexible Sigmoidoscopy

The most promising strategy for reducing the burden of colorectal cancer is periodic screening. Flexible sigmoidoscopy has been widely recommended at intervals of 3 to 5 years because of its sensitivity for detecting early cancers and adenomas. This examination is believed to be a cost-effective intervention for family physicians.

In most series, the average depth of insertion of the long flexible sigmoidoscope ranged between 48 and 55 cm. It is felt that about 60% of all colorectal cancers are within reach of the sigmoidoscope. The 3- to 5-year screening interval recommendation is based, in part, on the estimates of 7 to 10 years for an adenoma to progress to malignancy. Most organizations recommend initiating sigmoidoscopy screening at age 50 for individuals of average risk.

An important limitation to the effectiveness of screening for colorectal cancer is the ability of patients and clinicians to comply with testing. Flexible fiberoptic sigmoidoscopy is considered by many patients to be uncomfortable, embarrassing, and expensive, and they may be reluctant to agree to the testing. Studies of populations that are repeatedly advised to undergo sigmoidoscopy have found that only 10 to 30% of individuals agree to the procedure. Physician motivation is important in encouraging patient compliance for undergoing the procedure. Physicians report that the lengthy procedure time and the extensive training needed to master the technique limit their use of the sigmoidoscope. Once a physician becomes experienced in endoscopic techniques, however, sigmoidoscopy procedures can be performed routinely in less than 10 minutes.

METHODS AND MATERIALS

Patient Preparation

Confirm that the patient performed the recommended enemas and preparation. The patient should remove clothing from below the waistline, and should be seated on the examination table with a disposable sheet draped over the legs. Place an absorbent sheet beneath the patient on the table.

Equipment

Nonsterile Tray

Place the following items on a nonsterile drape covering on a Mayo stand:

> 2 or 3 nonsterile gloves (some physicians double-glove the right hand and remove the outer glove after the rectal examination and anoscopy)
>
> 1 inch of 4 × 4 gauze
>
> 1 inch of water-soluble (K-Y) jelly dispensed on one corner of the drape
>
> 1 inch of 5% lidocaine ointment dispensed on one corner of the drape
>
> An emesis basin filled with water for suction at the end of the procedure
>
> Ives anoscope

Endoscopy Cart

> Water bottle filled and connected to the light source
>
> Suction unit plugged into the wall outlet, and connected to the scope
>
> Light source plugged into the wall outlet, and the sigmoidoscope is connected to the light source.
>
> The operation of the sigmoidoscope should be checked before the procedure: air should be bubbled into the basin of water, and some of the water suctioned through.
>
> Biopsy forceps should be available (if in sterile packaging, do not open unless the forceps are needed).

PROCEDURE DESCRIPTION

1. The patient is placed in the left lateral decubitus position. A rectal examination is performed with the gloved finger, examining the prostate in the male patient, and confirming anal patency. The gloved examining finger can be lubricated with 2% lidocaine jelly (Lidocaine) or 5% lidocaine ointment to provide topical anesthesia of the anal canal for anoscope and sigmoidoscope insertion.
2. The lubricated slotted Ives anoscope is lubricated with water-soluble (K-Y) jelly or additional lidocaine jelly, and inserted into the anal canal. The three hemorrhoid pads (right posterior, right anterior, and left lateral) should be inspected individually, necessitating insertion of the scope three times, to examine for anal canal pathology.
3. The distal portion of the flexible sigmoidoscope is lubricated with water-soluble jelly, but the jelly is kept off the most distal tip to avoid smearing the lens and distorting the image. The scope is inserted into the rectum, either by direct insertion into the anus, or by pushing the scope tip into the anus by flexing the index finger behind the scope.
4. Once the scope is in the rectum (7 to 15 cm inserted), air is insufflated, fluid that may be present is suctioned, and the lumen is located by moving

the tip of the scope. While some examiners have the nurse or assistant insert the scope, better control of the scope tip is achieved if the right hand inserts the scope and rotates the tip to the right and left. The examiner's left thumb moves the scope tip up and down by moving the inner knob on the scope head.

5. The scope is inserted only while the lumen is visualized. Attempt to insert the scope as quickly as possible, thereby limiting patient discomfort. Special insertion techniques, such as torquing (twisting the scope in the right hand), dithering (rapid, short back and forth motions to advance the scope), or accordionization (pulling back on angled portions of colon wall with the scope tip, allowing the scope tip then to advance with the colon folded—like an accordion—onto the scope), and hooking and straightening (Fig. 4.1), may be required to negotiate the many turns in the sigmoid. The colon mucosa is inspected as the scope is withdrawn, and biopsies are obtained only if needed.

6. Once the scope tip is withdrawn to the rectum (10 to 15 cm inserted), the scope tip is retroverted to examine the distal rectal vault. This area is not seen well by the forward directed scope as it is either inserted or withdrawn. Retroversion is achieved by maximally deflecting the inner knob with the left thumb while simultaneously inserting the scope with the right hand. This maneuver should produce an image of the black scope as it enters the rectum from the anal canal.

7. Air is withdrawn from the rectum prior to removing the scope. The scope is immediately immersed in a basin of water, and the suction channel is flushed to prevent clogging of this channel by stool that may have entered the channel during the procedure. The anus is wiped clear with gauze, and the patient is offered the opportunity to go to the bathroom. Once the patient is dressed, the patient can be moved to a chair for postprocedure counseling while the scope is cleaned and disinfected.

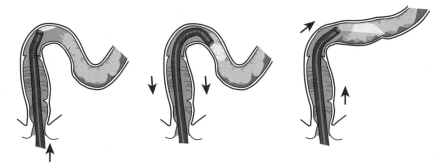

FIGURE 4.1. The hooking and straightening technique is used to pass through a tortuous sigmoid colon. The scope is inserted to the angled sigmoid, the scope tip is turned to a sharp angle, and the sigmoid is hooked as the scope is withdrawn. The sigmoid is straightened as the scope is withdrawn, and the scope can be inserted through to the descending colon.

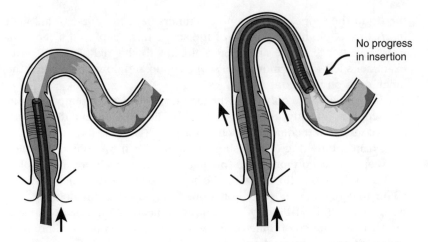

No progress
in insertion

FIGURE 4.2.   Paradoxical insertion describes the insertion of the tube without advancement of the scope tip. The scope is bowing out the sigmoid colon, which has a mobile mesenteric attachment. Paradoxical insertion can be very uncomfortable for the patient.

ANATOMY AND PATHOLOGY RECOGNITION DURING SIGMOIDOSCOPY

1. As the scope is inserted into the rectum, a red-out may develop if the scope tip is pushed up against the colon wall. The scope tip can be slowly withdrawn and air inserted until the lumen appears. The normal rectal mucosa demonstrates a nonfriable vascular network. Proctitis produces an erythematous, friable mucosa, often with bleeding. Preprocedure enemas given to clear the colon may produce some patchy or streaky erythema, which should not be confused with proctitis.

2. The semilunar valves of Houston generally appear as sharp edges protruding into the lumen, with dark shadows noted behind. These valves protrude from different sides of the rectum, and are more easily seen with air insufflation or when the scope is withdrawn on exiting the colon. The physician should examine for pathology behind the valves. Ulcerative colitis usually produces erythema, friability, and mucosal bleeding, which may extend from the anus upward throughout the colon.

3. As the scope enters the sigmoid, redundant folds (with a loss of vascularity) obliterate the lumen. Air insufflation is necessary to identify the lumen. Extensive turning of the scope tip, torquing, accordionization, or dithering techniques may be needed to negotiate the marked sigmoid turns. The examiner should avoid bowing out the sigmoid, which happens when the midscope is inserted into a sigmoid loop, but the scope tip fails to advance (Fig. 4.2).

4. The descending colon appears as a long tube ringed with concentric

haustrae. The vascularity of the descending colon appears as a random reticular pattern. Diverticular openings may be seen here, appearing as dark circles in the colon wall. Polyps may appear as a mound in the mucosa (sessile) or on a long stalk (pedunculated). Because mucus adherent to the colon wall can be mistaken for a sessile polyp, bulges in the wall can be tapped with the scope tip to see if they wipe off. Colon cancers can often be recognized by the irregular growth or mucosal pattern, bleeding or narrowing of the lumen.

5. The splenic flexure sometimes can be reached with the 60 cm sigmoidoscope. The splenic flexure can appear as a dead-end, and if the turn is negotiated, the triangular shape to the transverse colon may be visualized. Crohn's disease can produce mucosal cobblestoning, friability, and "skip areas" with normal mucosa separating areas of erythematous or diseased colon.

6. The last area to be visualized as the scope is withdrawn is the rectal vault. Because the lateral portions of the distal rectum are not well visualized by the forwardly directed scope, the scope tip can be retroverted. The scope is seen entering the rectum from the anal canal, and the upper extent of internal hemorrhoids can be identified.

TABLE 4.1. CPT Codes for Flexible Sigmoidoscopy

CPT Codes	Description	1998 Total RVUs[a]	1998 Average 50% Fees in U.S.[b]
45330	Flexible sigmoidoscopy [separate procedure]	2.31	$213
45331	Flexible sigmoidoscopy with biopsy, single or multiple	3.02	$268

CPT only © 1998 American Medical Association. All rights reserved.

[a]Department of Health and Human Services, Health Care Financing Administration. Medicare program: revisions to payment policies and adjustments to the relative value units (RVUs) under the physician fee schedule for calendar year 1998. Federal Register 42 CFR part 414. October 31, 1997;62(211):59103–59255.

[b]1998 Physicians' Fee Reference. West Allis, WI: Yale Wasserman, DMD, Medical Publishers, 1998.

FOLLOW UP

- Diminutive polyps (less than 5 mm in diameter) cannot be classified by visual inspection. All polyps less than 5 mm should have biopsies performed. If the polyp is hyperplastic, no further treatment is necessary, since hyperplastic polyps are not associated with polyps in the proximal (right) colon. If the polyp is adenomatous (tubular, villous, etc.) then a full colonoscopy should be performed to look for synchronous proximal polyps.
- Larger polyps (greater than 5 to 10 mm in diameter) generally are adenomatous and do not require a biopsy at sigmoidoscopy because they should

be completely removed. Polypectomy is performed during colonoscopy to facilitate the search for any additional polyps.

- If a suspected cancer is encountered (an irregular, obstructing, friable, or bleeding mass), the patient can have a biopsy performed, but vigorous bleeding of the lesion may ensue. Prompt referral is suggested.
- Diverticulosis is believed to result from the colon's exposure to excessive intraluminal pressure. Patients with diverticulosis can be offered stool bulking agents to soften the stools and to reduce stool transit time. Patients with diverticulosis are often told to avoid nuts and seeds in their diet to prevent an undigested seed from clogging a diverticular opening, although there is little evidence suggesting this.
- Hemorrhoids are commonly encountered during sigmoidoscopy. Surgical or ablative therapies can be considered, but the hemorrhoids often shrink with administration of stool-bulking agents and efforts to promote soft stools.
- Nonspecific colitis is a frequent finding with many causes. While multiple biopsies are recommended, they often cannot identify the etiology of the colitis, or distinguish Crohn's disease from ulcerative colitis. Referral can be made, although some physicians may consider empiric treatment with salicylate-based anti-inflammatory medications or hydrocortisone enemas.
- Pseudomembranes may be encountered in a patient with diarrhea. A recent history of antibiotic use should be sought, and endoscopic brushings or stool samples for *Clostridium difficile* can confirm the diagnosis. Treatment with vancomycin (Vancocin) or metronidazole (Flagyl) may be considered.

PROCEDURE PITFALLS/COMPLICATIONS

- *The image frequently appears as a red-out.* When the scope tip is up against the colon wall, the image becomes blurred into a red-out. Whenever a red-out is encountered, additional air can be insufflated and the scope tip should be withdrawn until the lumen is relocated.

- *The patient complains of severe pain during the examination.* Discomfort during the examination results from several factors, including the insertion technique. Overinflation of the colon with air can cause discomfort, sweating, and a vagal response. Lengthy procedure times also produce discomfort. Physicians should strive to limit the insertion time to 5 minutes, with more time used to examine the colon on withdrawal of the scope. Premedication with diazepam or triazolam can be considered for anxious patients, and the patient's back can be rubbed by the nurse or assistant during the most uncomfortable parts of the examination.

- *The scope tip doesn't seem to advance when inserted.* The sigmoid portion of the colon can be bowed out with scope insertion, often with no advancement of the scope tip. This sigmoid bowing, however, can produce significant discomfort. When insertion of the scope fails to advance the tip, consider twisting or torquing the scope to effectively provide more rigidity to the flexible distal portion of the scope to facilitate insertion.

- *The slide-by technique to pass through the sigmoid involves some risk.* The slide-by technique inserts the scope by pushing the scope tip along the colon wall. This technique involves some risk. By pressing the scope against the colon wall, tears and bleeding can occur in the mesentery supporting the colon. Perforations may be more common when the slide-by technique is used. Many experts strongly recommend insertion of the scope only when the lumen can be visualized.

- *Retroversion of the scope tip at the end of the procedure seems unnecessary.* Retroverting the scope tip allows for visualization of the lateral portions of the distal rectum. Because this area is not seen well by the forward-directed scope, small polyps or cancers can fail to be detected unless retroversion is performed.

- *A diverticular opening is large enough to allow for insertion of the scope tip.* Occasionally diverticular openings are so large that they can be mistaken for the colon lumen. Because diverticula have very thin walls, entering a diverticula can easily lead to a perforation. Acute diverticulitis can produce an erythematous, swollen, or bleeding diverticular opening. Sliding the scope past an acutely inflamed diverticular opening can result in significant complications. If such an opening is encountered, the scope should be immediately withdrawn.

- *Inflammatory bowel disease cannot be definitively diagnosed visually.* Colitis can result from many causes including infection, autoimmune disorders, and medications. The diagnosis may not be apparent from the visual appearance of the colon, and biopsies can help to identify the cause of colitis. Biopsies, however, may not be able to differentiate Crohn's disease form ulcerative colitis.

- *The patient requests that the endoscopy be terminated early in the procedure.* Scope insertion should not continue against the patient's wishes. Legal concerns over the disregard for the patient's rights make it imperative that physicians not advance the scope over the objections of the patient.

PHYSICIAN TRAINING

Physicians can benefit from a comprehensive course on sigmoidoscopy, such as the one offered by the American Academy of Family Physicians. Physicians need to be well versed in pathology recognition, and many good atlases can be consulted for this. Physicians can practice the manual skills of scope manipulation on models. Great debate exists over the minimum number of procedures needed for competency. Gastroenterology organizations have suggested procedure numbers of 25 to 100 before privileges be granted. Many physicians have demonstrated good skills after just 10 procedures. Physicians should strive to have as many supervised procedures as they need to be comfortable with scope insertion and pathology recognition. Most physicians achieve comfort after 10 to 25 procedures. Unsupervised procedures should not be performed unless the physician has had some precepted experience.

ORDERING INFORMATION

Flexible sigmoidoscope, light source, water bottle, biopsy forceps, cleaning materials (Olympus OSF, Olympus Corporation, 4 Nevada Drive, Lake Success, NY; 516-488-3880)

Ives anoscope (Redfield Corporation, 210 Summit Avenue, Montvale, NJ; 800-678-4472)

K-Y lubricating jelly (4 oz. tube, Johnson & Johnson Medical, Arlington, TX; 800-443-5009)

5% lidocaine ointment (3.5 g tube, Astra, Westborough, MA; 508-366-1100)

BIBLIOGRAPHY

American Academy of Family Physicians. Flexible sigmoidoscopy preceptorial training program: a syllabus for the physician starting to perform flexible sigmoidoscopy in the office. Kansas City: AAFP, 1985.

Cohen LB. A new illustrated 'how to' guide to flexible sigmoidoscopy. Prim Care Cancer 1989;9:13-20.

Coller JA. Technique of flexible fiberoptic sigmoidoscopy. Surg Clin North Am 1980;60:465-479.

Hocutt JE, Jaffe R, Owens GM, Walters DT. Flexible fiberoptic sigmoidoscopy. Am Fam Physician 1982;26:133-141.

Neugut AI, Pita S. Role of sigmoidoscopy in screening for colorectal cancer: a critical review. Gastroenterology 1988;95:492-499.

Ransohoff DF, Lang CA. Sigmoidoscopic screening in the 1990s. JAMA 1993;269:1278-1281.

Rees MK. We should all be performing flexible sigmoidoscopy. Modern Med 1987;55:3,12.

Rodney WM. Procedural skills in flexible sigmoidoscopy and colonoscopy for the family physician. Primary Care 1988;15:79-91.

Williams JJ. Why family physicians should perform sigmoidoscopy [Editorial]. Am Fam Physician 1990;4:1722,1724.

Winawer SJ. Office screening for colorectal cancer. Prim Care Cancer 1993;13:37-46.

CHAPTER 5

. . . .

Lumbar Puncture

The examination of the cerebrospinal fluid historically has been a mainstay of neurologic diagnosis. Although lumbar puncture has several therapeutic uses, its greatest value is as a diagnostic test. Because of the diagnostic limitations of the test and the risks associated with the procedure, however, decisions to perform lumbar puncture must be made carefully.

Lumbar puncture is potentially useful for diagnosing or excluding conditions that involve the meninges or produce changes in the cerebrospinal fluid (CSF) caused by alterations in the blood-brain barrier (Table 5.1). The four major classes of disease diagnosed by lumbar puncture include: meningeal infection, subarachnoid hemorrhage, central nervous system malignancy, and demyelinating disease. Historically, patients with dementia have undergone lumbar puncture primarily to exclude neurosyphilis or cryptococcal meningitis. It is currently believed that in the great majority of patients with dementia, evaluation of the CSF fails to provide information contributing to a specific cause.

The indications for lumbar puncture in the newborn are not as clear as once believed. There is considerable doubt regarding the clinical utility of performing the test in all ill newborns with suspected sepsis or respiratory distress, unless other findings suggest meningitis. Some authors have advocated that lumbar puncture be reserved for those babies who demonstrate hypothermia, hyperthermia, poor feeding beyond 24 hours of age, coma, or seizures. Lumbar puncture for the diagnosis of intracranial hemorrhage is rarely needed with the introduction of bedside ultrasound scanning. Traumatic (bloody) taps and unsuccessful taps are common in newborns, with only half of all taps successfully completed. Epidermoid spinal cord tumors have been associated with the performance of lumbar puncture in infants with unstyletted needles.

While lumbar puncture is considered relatively safe, complications range from mild discomfort to fatal reactions (Table 5.2). Headache is the most common complication (5 to 25%), often persisting for days. Using smaller diameter needles, providing adequate hydration, and keeping the patient supine or (even better) prone following the procedure can reduce this complication.

METHODS AND MATERIALS

Patient Preparation

Proper positioning of the patient and needle are critical for obtaining adequate amounts of CSF. The patient is curled into the lateral decubitus position with the back positioned at the edge of the table. The vertical plane of the back should be perpendicular to the table. The needle is inserted in the midline, with frequent removal of the stylet to determine when the needle tip has entered the subarachnoid space.

Equipment

Most physicians use a purchased sterile lumbar puncture tray that contains the following items:

18-gauge 3½-inch spinal needle

22-gauge 1½-inch infiltration needle

25-gauge ⅝-inch infiltration needle

Three-way stopcock

Manometer (2-piece)

Extension tubing

4 numbered specimen tubes (10 mL)

2×2-inch gauze

3 handled skin cleansing sponges

Lidocaine 1% (2 mL) (Xylocaine)

Bandage

TABLE 5.1. Indications for Lumbar Puncture

Evaluation/Diagnosis

Infectious diseases/meningitis
Central nervous system syphilis
Subarachnoid hemorrhage
Central nervous system malignancy
Multiple sclerosis
Guillain-Barré syndrome
Neonate with neurologic symptoms or signs

Therapeutic Uses

Intrathecal administration of antineoplastic or other medications
Serial removal of CSF

TABLE 5.2. Complications of Lumbar Puncture

Headache
Nerve injury
Painful paresthesias in the legs
Persisting pain or paresthesias following the procedure
Spinal hematoma
Brain herniation and death
Spinal infection
Local pain in the back

Towel

Fenestrated drape

Povidone-iodine solution (must be poured into one of the empty plastic wells on the tray after the tray is opened, being careful to avoid contaminating the tray contents)

Sterile gloves for the physician

PROCEDURE TECHNIQUE

1. The patient can be seated facing the back of an upright chair, or placed in the left lateral decubitus position. If lying in the lateral position, the hips, knees, and neck are flexed toward the abdomen and the back is kept vertical and placed at the edge of the table. An assistant can help the patient maintain this position throughout the procedure. The tops of the iliac crests are palpated bilaterally, and the L3–L4 interspace is identified just below the imaginary line that joins the tops of the iliac crests (Fig. 5.1). Some physicians create a pressure mark (with their fingernail) in the skin to mark the midline needle insertion site between vertebral processes.

2. The lumbar puncture tray is opened and the physician puts on the sterile gloves. The manometer/stopcock/pressure measurement tubing is assembled. Four specimen containers are opened and placed upright in their holding slots. The 1% lidocaine is drawn into the 3 mL syringe. The assistant pours povidone-iodine solution into one of the sterile wells.

3. The handled cleaning sponges are used to cleanse the skin with povidone-iodine solution, starting at the intended needle insertion site and progressing outward in enlarging circles. The fenestrated drape is placed, applying the adhesive strips onto the patient once the fenestration (hole) is centered over the needle insertion site. The sterile gloves should not be contaminated during drape placement.

4. The landmarks are palpated again through the drape, and the intended

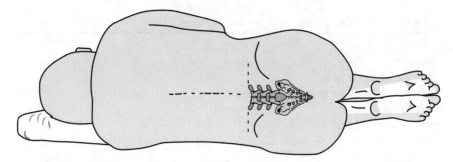

FIGURE 5.1.   The L3–L4 interspace is identified just below the imaginary line that joins the tops of the iliac crest.

needle insertion site confirmed. The anesthetic is administered in the skin, beneath the skin, and deep into the interspinous ligament near the dura. The spinal needle and stylet are then inserted into the anesthetized skin and between the vertebral spinous processes. The needle must be maintained in the midline. The needle can be angled 20° cephalad, aiming toward the umbilicus, to facilitate entry into the subarachnoid space. Some authors advocate turning the bevel of the needle parallel to the table, so the needle tip separates, rather than transects, the nerves of the cauda equina.

5. The needle insertion should proceed steadily, but cautiously. After the needle is inserted about 1 to 1½ inch, the stylet can be removed to check for fluid. If the needle is not inserted deep enough, dark blood from the prespinal venous plexus overlying the dura will fill the needle. Usually a "pop" or "give" will be felt as the needle penetrates the dura. Once the dura has been penetrated, clear spinal fluid usually flows freely. If the needle tip comes up against bone, the needle can be partially withdrawn and the insertion angle slightly altered to penetrate the subarachnoid space. If the patient has arthritis or spurs, the needle can be "walked" down the bone to find an opening.

6. Once clear fluid is noted in the needle, the examiner's thumb is placed over the hub of the needle to limit spillage. The stopcock and manometer are attached gently to the needle hub, with care not to move the spinal needle's position. An opening pressure reading can be obtained. Some authors advocate straightening the patient's legs and getting the patient to relax to obtain a more accurate opening pressure. The opening pressure reading is the site where the column of fluid fails to rise (excluding respiratory variations). A normal opening pressure is less than 20 mmHg, and elevated pressures are above 25 mm Hg. The stopcock can be turned to allow the fluid in the manometer to be collected in tube 1. The stopcock and manometer are placed back on the tray, and the tubes are

successively filled directly from the needle hub with 0.5 to 3 mL of fluid. For an adult, 2 mL in each tube is usually adequate.

7. Once the collection tubes are filled, the stylet is reinserted inside the needle. The needle is withdrawn, and immediate pressure is applied to the site with 2×2 inch gauze. Some authors advise rubbing the skin site for 15 to 30 seconds to produce local swelling and reduce the likelihood of a persisting dural leak into the needle tract and a postprocedure headache.

8. The povidone-iodine solution is wiped off the skin and a bandage is applied. The patient is encouraged to lay flat (supine or prone) for at least 4 hours following the procedure.

9. The collections tubes are sent for analysis (Table 5.3).

FOLLOW-UP

See Tables 5.3 and 5.4.

TABLE 5.3.   Spinal Fluid Testing

Recommended Initial Battery of Tests

Tube 1 Glucose and protein
Tube 2 Gram stain and culture and sensitivity
Tube 3 Cell count and differential
Tube 4 Most authors advocate holding the fluid in the fourth tube for additional studies should they be needed.

Additional Tests That Are Commonly Performed

KOH
Fungal cultures
AFB smears
Tb cultures
VDRL
Protein electrophoresis
Cytological examination
Oligoclonal banding

PROCEDURE PITFALLS/COMPLICATIONS

• *Firm resistance is noted when the needle is inserted.* If firm resistance is encountered with needle insertion, the needle is probably up against the underlying bone. The needle should be withdrawn and redirected until it enters the subarachnoid space. If the needle encounters bone, the needle tip can be "walked down the bone," or incrementally moved in one direction until the bony obstruction is cleared.

- *The patient complains of radiating pain down the leg during insertion.* If the patient complains of radiating pain down a lower extremity, a nerve root of the cauda equina probably has been struck. The procedure can continue; the floating nerve usually is pushed aside and not damaged by the advancing needle. Never try to aspirate spinal fluid during the procedure, as the nerve roots can be suctioned into the needle and the nerves traumatized.

- *Epidermoid spinal tumors have been noted after use of butterfly needles in infants.* Because of the large, cumbersome spinal needles that are used in infants, several variations in technique have been advocated. The author of this book advocates only the use of styletted needles. Use caution when performing lumbar puncture in infants using unstyletted needles, such as butterfly needles, since epidermoid spinal tumors have been noted many years following this technique.

- *A brain herniation from elevated intracranial pressure followed the lumbar puncture.* Herniation frequently results in death, and is the most feared consequence of lumbar puncture. This complication usually happens with increased intracranial pressure. One large study of lumbar puncture in patients with increased intracranial pressure demonstrated that herniation occurs in 1% of patients with papilledema, but in 12% of patients without papilledema. Lumbar puncture should be approached cautiously in patients known to have increased intracranial pressure.

- *Most of my taps are bloody.* The traumatic tap occurs in 20% of adult patients undergoing lumbar puncture. Bloody taps often occur because of inadvertent puncture of the venous plexuses located dorsally and ventrally to the spinal sack, or to injury to the vessels that accompany the cauda equina. This bleeding rarely causes harm to the patient. The majority of bleeding comes from the dorsal plexus, with inadequate needle insertion. Continued midline insertion of the needle until the "give" or "pop" of entry into the subarachnoid space can reduce bloody taps.

- *Death followed lumbar puncture in a very ill infant.* While lumbar puncture has been considered mandatory in the evaluation of children with suspected meningitis, some children deteriorate or even die following the procedure. The procedure may be too risky in children showing signs of increased intracranial pressure. Such signs could include deterioration of the level of consciousness, decerebrate or decorticate rigidity, tonic seizures, unilateral or bilateral fixed pupils, loss or paresis of ocular movements, hemiparesis, apnea or irregular respiration, and extensor plantar responses.

TABLE 5.4. Characteristics of CSF in Various Conditions

Condition	Cell Count	Glucose	Other
Bacterial meningitis	500–10,000 WBCs with 90–95% PMNs	0–40	Gram stain positive in 70–80% Culture positive in 80–90%
Tuberculous meningitis	25–500 WBCs with >80% lympho-cytes	10–40	PMNs can predominate early
Viral meningitis	6–1000 WBCs	Normal (60% of blood glucose)	—
Syphilitic meningitis	100–500 WBCs	Normal or decreased	Reagin or treponemal tests positive
Seizure disorder	0–500 WBCs	Normal	CSF pleocytosis may result from seizures
Traumatic tap	Increased RBCs, xan-thochromia, clot-ting of bloody fluid	Normal or elevated	Clearing of RBCs from CSF from tube 1 to 4
Multiple sclerosis	0–20 lymphocytes	Normal	Elev. CSF Ig G in 66% Oligoclonal bands in 90%
Guillain-Barré syndrome	Cell count usually normal 15% have 10–215 lymphocytes	Normal	Protein up to 1000 mg/dl CSF protein rise after 1–2 wks.
Subarachnoid hemor-rhage	1000–3.5 million RBCs	Normal Low in 10%	Protein elevation from serum protein
Meningeal carcinoma-tosis	10–500 WBCs, pre-dominately lym-phocytes	Below 40	False-negative cytology in 9%

TABLE 5.5. CPT Codes for Lumbar Puncture

CPT Codes	Description	1998 Total RVUs[a]	1998 Average 50% Fees in U.S.[b]
62270	Diagnostic lumbar puncture	1.90	$165
62272	Therapeutic (drainage) lumbar puncture	2.48	$205

[a] Department of Health and Human Services, Health Care Financing Administration. Medicare program: revisions to payment policies and adjustments to the relative value units (RVUs) under the physician fee schedule for calendar year 1998. Federal Register 42 CFR part 414. October 31, 1997; 62(211);59103–59255.

[b] 1998 Physicians' Fee Reference. West Allis, WI: Yale Wasserman, DMD, Medical Publishers, 1998.

PHYSICIAN TRAINING

While the technique of lumbar puncture is easy to learn, mastering the needle manipulation with minimal patient discomfort requires some experience. There is a significant rate of unsuccessful lumbar puncture procedures, especially when performed on neonates. It is probably safe for physicians to perform unsupervised lumbar puncture procedures after three to five supervised procedures; however, since experience can assist the physician in refining techniques used in lumbar puncture, physicians should strive to perform at least 10 supervised procedures in both adults and children.

ORDERING INFORMATION

Lumbar Puncture Tray (Baxter Healthcare Corporation, 1 Baxter Parkway, Deerfield, IL 60015; 800-933-0303)

BIBLIOGRAPHY

Addy DP. When not to do a lumbar puncture. Arch Dis Child 1987;62:873–875.

Eng RKH, Seligman SJ. Lumbar puncture-induced meningitis. JAMA 1981;245:1456–1459.

Gilland O. How to take the headache out of spinal taps. Headache 1969;9:154–158.

Gorelick PB, Biller J. Lumbar puncture: techniques, indications and complications. Postgrad Med 1986;79:257–268.

Halcrow SJ, Crawford PJ, Craft AW. Epidermoid spinal cord tumour after lumbar puncture. Arch Dis Child 1985;60:978–979.

Halliday HL. When to do a lumbar puncture in a neonate. Arch Dis Child 1989;64:313–316.

Hildebrand WL, Stevens DC, Gosling CG, Sternecker CL, Schreiner RL. Lumbar puncture in infants. Am Fam Phys 1983;27:157–159.

Marton KI, Gean AD. The spinal tap: a new look at an old test. Ann Intern Med 1986;104:840–848.

Morgenlander JC. Lumbar puncture and CSF examination. Postgrad Med 1994;95:125–131.

Raskin NH. Lumbar puncture headache: a review. Headache 1990;30:197–200.

CHAPTER 6

Flexible Nasolaryngoscopy

The flexible fiberoptic nasolaryngoscope has become a valuable diagnostic tool for family physicians in the diagnosis and management of conditions affecting the upper respiratory tract. The technique of nasolaryngoscopy is easily learned, and is a cost-effective means of viewing an area that had previously been hidden.

Nasolaryngoscopy provides a much more complete and accurate examination than older, indirect-viewing techniques, and leads to improved diagnosis and improved management of many common head and neck complaints (Table 6.1). In one large series of family practice patients, 70% of patients had a change in the management plan after nasolaryngoscopy.

Nasolaryngoscopy is well-tolerated by both adults and children. Patients appreciate the reassurance this technique can provide, especially when performed in the convenience and familiar environment of their family physician's office. Contraindications to the procedure include an uncooperative patient, epiglottitis, or active epistaxis. Complications are rare and are generally minimal in nature.

METHODS AND MATERIALS

Patient Preparation

The patient is seated on an electric table, and the upper portion of the table is raised to support the patient's back. The entire table is raised to place the patient's head at (or just below) the height of the examiner's head. The patient is given tissues for one hand, and an emesis basin to hold in the other hand. An adsorbent sheet is draped over the shoulders and tucked inside the patient's collar.

Equipment

Place the following items on a drape covering the Mayo stand:

2% lidocaine jelly

Bottle of oxymetazoline hydrochloride 0.05% (Afrin) spray

4% lidocaine solution in an atomizer spray bottle

1 inch of nonsterile 4×4 gauze

TABLE 6.1. Procedure Indications

Acid (reflux) laryngitis
Chronic cough
Chronic halitosis
Chronic hoarseness (persisting more than 3 weeks)
Chronic nasal obstruction
Chronic pharyngeal pain
Chronic postnasal drainage
Chronic rhinorrhea
Chronic serous otitis media in an adult
Chronic sinus discomfort
Chronic sinusitis
Dysphagia
Follow up after conservative treatment of laryngeal polyps
Follow up of previous radiation therapy or surgical procedures
Foreign body sensation in the pharynx
Globus hystericus
Hemoptysis
Laryngeal mass
Prior history of head or neck cancer
Prolonged acid reflux
Recurrent epistaxis
Recurrent Eustachian tube dysfunction
Recurrent otalgia
Suspected foreign body
Suspected nasal polyps
Suspected neoplasm
Vocal cord inflammation
Vocal cord nodules
Vocal cord paralysis

Flexible fiberoptic nasolaryngoscope (3.5 mm outer diameter) attached to the light source

Suction machine should be available if needed

Endoscope sterilization equipment

PROCEDURE DESCRIPTION

1. The patient is placed in a seated position, with the chin slightly forward (as if sniffing flowers). It is best if the procedure is performed with the patient on an electric table so that the patient's head can be adjusted

to just below or at the same height as the examiner's head. If an electric table is not available, the back of an exam table should be raised so the patient's head is at the same height as the examiner's. An absorbent sheet is draped over the patient's shoulders and tucked inside the patient's collar. The patient is given a few tissues to hold in one hand, and a plastic emesis basin to hold in the other.

2. The patient receives two sprays of the decongestant oxymetazoline hydrochloride 0.05% in each nostril to increase the available space for passage of the scope. The spray nozzle of the bottle is held just outside the patient's nostril and does not touch the patient so that it can be used again.

3. The patient's nose is then sprayed with 4% lidocaine solution through an atomizer. The solution has a sour taste, and the patient should be warned. The examiner should pause for a few seconds after the initial sprays are administered, allowing the patient time to recover and for the medication to take effect. Repeat the sprays until both sides of the nose and the larynx are adequately anesthetized (i.e., the patient reports lack of sensation in the back of the throat).

4. The flexible fiberoptic scope is held in the left hand, with the eyepiece pointing up, and the scope tip pointing to the floor. The scope should be traversing the palmar creases of the examiner's left hand. The up and down control knob is moved with the left thumb, and the right and left turning is performed by twisting the scope tip side to side with the first two fingers of the right hand.

5. The distal portion of the scope is lubricated with 2% lidocaine jelly. The jelly never is applied to the scope tip, as this will blur the view. The scope tip is grasped with the gloved right hand's first and second fingertips. If the scope is too slippery, use a piece of 4×4 gauze held with the first two fingers.

6. The scope tip is gently inserted into the nares. The right first two fingers should insert and turn the scope, while the right third, fourth, and fifth fingers gently rest on the patient's cheek like a tripod. These fingers provide contact with the patient, stabilizing the examiner's hand in the event of sudden patient movement. Warn the patient of a tickling sensation as the scope enters the nose.

7. The floor of the nose, or inferior meatus (area beneath the inferior turbinate), is usually the largest passage to the nasopharynx. The nasopharynx is completely examined, turning the scope to view the eustachian tube opening and torus tubarius on each side.

8. The scope tip is deflected down, and the larynx is seen in the distance. The scope is slowly advanced to just above the epiglottis. Touching the pharynx walls or laryngeal structures can induce coughing or gagging and, therefore, should be avoided.

9. The larynx is thoroughly evaluated, with the scope tip always kept above

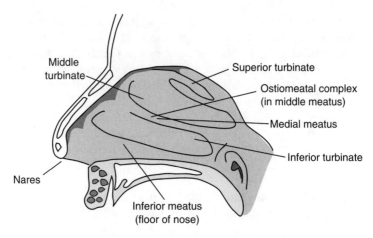

FIGURE 6.1. Left nasal cavity.

the level of the vocal cords (to avoid laryngospasm). Ask the patient to say "E" as the pitch of the voice is increased, watching the movement of the vocal cords. The patient can assist in viewing the vallecula by protruding the tongue.

10. The scope tip is returned to the nasopharynx. The scope tip should be directed up, to view the sphenoid sinus ostia. This area does not receive the anesthetic spray, and the patient must be warned about the discomfort that frequently accompanies this maneuver.

11. The scope tip is returned to the nasopharynx, and this area is reexamined. The scope is withdrawn to where the tip lies in the middle of the inferior meatus. The tip is elevated to the level of the middle meatus, just below the middle turbinate.

12. The middle meatus may be anatomically narrow, and this maneuver may be uncomfortable for the patient. Attempt to visualize the infundibulum area (osteomeatal complex) and the maxillary sinus ostia, although even the most experienced endoscopists often cannot adequately view these structures.

13. The scope is withdrawn, and the drape removed. The patient may wish to blow his or her nose. The physician reviews the findings with the patient.

ANATOMIC SITES VISUALIZED

Nose (Fig. 6.1): inferior turbinate, inferior meatus, middle turbinate, middle meatus, superior turbinate, medial crura of the lower septal cartilage, maxillary sinus ostia, frontal sinus ostia, sphenoid sinus ostia, infundibulum (osteomeatal complex), septum

Nasopharynx (Fig. 6.2): right torus tubarius, left torus tubarius, right Eustachian tube ostia, left Eustachian tube ostia, right adenoid pad, left adenoid pad, right Rosenmüller's fossa, left Rosenmüller's fossa, superior aspect of the soft palate

Hypopharynx: lingual tonsils, palatine tonsils, posterior tongue, posterior pharyngeal wall

Larynx (Fig. 6.3): epiglottis, vallecula, aryepiglottic folds, right piriform sinus, left piriform sinus, corniculate cartilages, cuneiform cartilages, true vocal cords, false vocal cords

COMMON PATHOLOGY ENCOUNTERED

Nose: abnormal vasculature, swollen turbinate mucosa, polyps, foreign body, purulent sinus drainage, deviated septum, hypertrophied turbinate, papillomas, septal perforation

Nasopharynx: purulent Eustachian tube drainage, adenoid hypertrophy, mucosa ulceration, nasopharyngeal cancer, abnormal vasculature

Hypopharynx: tonsillar hypertrophy, lymphoid hypertrophy of the tongue

Larynx: laryngeal polyps, laryngeal papillomas, laryngeal cancer, vocal cord leukoplakia, vocal cord (speaker's) nodules, acid laryngitis, vocal cord paralysis, vocal cord ulceration, foreign body

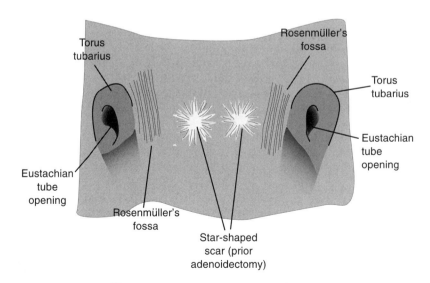

FIGURE 6.2. Posterior nasopharynx.

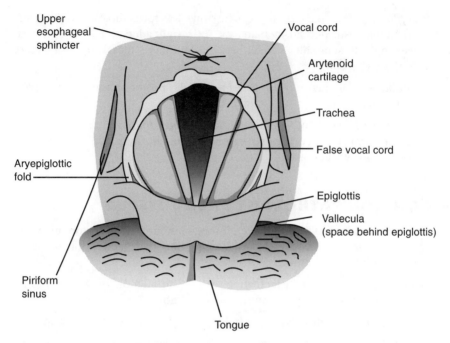

FIGURE 6.3. Larynx structures.

FOLLOW UP

- Unusual findings, tumors, or pathology that is unfamiliar to the examiner should be referred to an otolaryngologist or to a physician more experienced in upper respiratory disorders. Most diagnostic flexible laryngoscopes do not have the capability to biopsy. The performance of biopsies is usually best left to surgical specialists who can deal with the significant bleeding complications that may follow a biopsy.
- Acid laryngitis is a common finding at nasolaryngoscopy. The posterior larynx may appear erythematous, swollen, or inflamed. Suspected acid laryngitis or acid reflux swelling around the eustachian tube orifices can be empirically treated with an H_2 blocker or a proton pump inhibitor.
- Laryngeal cancer can produce subtle changes early in its course. The findings of vocal cord polyps, tumors, and other lesions should prompt a referral from the examiner when discovered.
- Nasal findings suggestive of allergic disease (swollen, pale, boggy turbinates) should prompt consideration for therapy. Steroid nasal sprays may be very effective in relieving symptoms.
- Some physicians will attempt to shrink small nasal polyps with steroid nasal sprays. Large polyps rarely resolve spontaneously, and often need surgical removal.

- Sinus drainage or pus is commonly encountered at nasolaryngoscopy. Therapy with antibiotics, decongestants, and anti-inflammatory nasal sprays may be beneficial.
- Adenoid hypertrophy, tonsillar hypertrophy, or lingual lymphoid tissue hypertrophy all can be considered for treatment with anti-inflammatory medications.
- Turbinate hypertrophy associated with nasal obstruction is commonly noted at nasolaryngoscopy. If patients with turbinate hypertrophy fail to respond to nasal steroid sprays, then they can be considered for turbinate reduction.

PROCEDURE PITFALLS/COMPLICATIONS

- ***When examining the nasopharynx, the view becomes blurry.*** Mucus can obscure the view during the examination. Instead of withdrawing the scope and starting over, ask the patient to swallow a few times, to produce a windshield wiper effect in clearing the scope tip. If this does not work, touch the scope tip to a side wall (as long as you are not in the larynx) to clear the mucus.

- ***The structures beneath the middle turbinate cannot be adequately visualized.*** Even expert examiners may be unable to negotiate the narrow area beneath the middle turbinate. Attempt to examine this area during every study, but physicians should not be frustrated if it cannot be visualized.

- ***The patient experiences excessive gagging when the larynx is examined.*** Care must be given to keep the scope off the walls of the hypopharynx, or to keep the scope tip from banging into the epiglottis or other structures of the larynx. Withdraw the tip of the scope to the nasopharynx if excessive gagging is encountered.

- ***The patient jerks during the procedure.*** The patient should be warned during the procedure of any maneuvers that may be uncomfortable, such as examination of the sphenoid sinus ostia. Maintain contact with the patient's face at all times by resting the right third, fourth, and fifth fingers against the cheek.

- ***The patient stops breathing when being examined below the cords.*** The scope tip should not be placed between or below the vocal cords during diagnostic nasolaryngoscopy examination. Laryngospasm is a potentially serious complication that can develop when the scope touches the structures of the larynx. Fortunately, most episodes of laryngospasm resolve without sequelae. If this complication occurs, the scope should immediately be withdrawn completely.

- ***Other potential complications.*** Gagging; vomiting; coughing; sneezing;

adverse reactions to the medications used during the procedure; discomfort; bleeding; and cardiovascular complications (rare), such as tachycardia or vasovagal reaction (bradycardia), are all potential complications.

TABLE 6.2. CPT Codes for Nasolaryngoscopy

CPT Codes[a]	Description	1998 Total RVUs[b]	1998 Average 50% Fees in U.S.[c]
31231	Diagnostic nasal endoscopy, unilateral or bilateral [separate procedure]	2.62	$198
31575	Diagnostic flexible fiberoptic laryngoscopy	2.83	$250
92511	Nasopharyngoscopy with endoscope [separate procedure]	1.78	$150

CPT only © 1998 American Medical Association. All rights reserved.
[a] Usually 31231 or 31575 is used to report the complete examination, although both codes are occasionally reported together. The single code that describes the area of main investigation is usually selected.
[b] Department of Health and Human Services, Health Care Financing Administration. Medicare program: revisions to payment policies and adjustments to the relative value units (RVUs) under the physician fee schedule for calendar year 1998. Federal Register 42 CFR part 414. October 31, 1997; 62(211):59103–59255.
[c] 1998 Physicians' Fee Reference. West Allis, WI: Yale Wasserman, DMD, Medical Publishers, 1998.

PHYSICIAN TRAINING

Physicians are urged to take a formal training course in this technique, such as the one offered by the American Academy of Family Physicians (AAFP). After the formal course, physicians should perform a number of supervised procedures with an experienced examiner. If a physician is experienced in other endoscopic procedures, the physician may be comfortable manipulating the scope after as few as three to five procedures. Other physicians may need 15 to 20 supervised procedures performing the procedure unassisted.

The most difficult aspect of nasolaryngoscopy is not scope manipulation, but maintaining familiarity with the complex anatomy of the nose and throat. Novice examiners often confuse normal anatomy for pathologic conditions. Atlases and videotapes are valuable teaching aids for physicians performing this procedure. Physicians who do not frequently perform this procedure can benefit from a brief review of the anatomy before each procedure.

EDUCATIONAL RESOURCES

The following videotapes are available free of charge from Glaxo Educational Resource Center (800-824-2896):

GVL 354 *Living Video Anatomy and Pathology in ENT: The Ear*

GVL 355 *Living Video Anatomy and Pathology in ENT: The Throat*

GVL 356 *Living Video Anatomy and Pathology in ENT: The Nose*

GVL 245 *Upper Airway Examination: Rhinoscopy*

The videotape *Current Concepts in Examination of the Nasopharynx and Larynx* can be obtained from the Pentax Continuing Education Library, Pentax Corporation, Orangeburg, NY 10962, 800-824-2896. There may be a charge for this videotape.

The AAFP also offers courses on nasolaryngoscopy and an instructional syllabus. Call the AAFP Order Department at 800-944-0000 for more information.

RECOMMENDED ATLASES

Becker W, et al. Atlas of ear, nose and throat diseases including bronchoesophagology. Philadelphia: WB Saunders, 1984.

Bull TR. Color atlas of ENT diagnosis. 2nd ed. St Louis: Wolfe Medical, 1987.

ORDERING INFORMATION

Lidocaine Hydrochloride 2% jelly (30-mL tube; Xylocaine jelly, Astra Pharmaceuticals, 50 Otis Street, Westborough, MA 01581; 508-366-1100, or through a local pharmacy)

Lidocaine hydrochloride 4% solution (50-mL bottle; Xylocaine 4% solution, Astra USA, Inc, 50 Otis Street, Westborough, MA 01581; 508-366-1100, or through a local pharmacy)

Nasolaryngoscope and light source (Welch Allyn RL-100, Welch Allyn, 4341 State Street, Skaneateles Falls, NY 13153; 800-535-6663, estimated cost for system: $5300)

Oxymetazoline HCl 0.05% (15-mL bottle; Afrin spray, Schering-Plough, 2000 Galloping Hill Road, Kenilworth, NJ 07033; 908-298-4000, or through a local pharmacy)

BIBLIOGRAPHY

Corey GA, Rodney WM, Hocutt JE. Rhinolaryngoscopy by family physicians. J Fam Pract 1990;31:49–52.

Curry RW. Flexible fiberoptic nasolaryngoscopy. Fam Pract Recert 1990;12:21–36.

DeWitt DE. Fiberoptic rhinolaryngoscopy in primary care. A new direction for expanding in-office diagnostics. Postgrad Med 1988;84(5):125–126, 131–135, 183.

Donnelly JP. The out-patient use of the fibrebronchoscope for examining the larynx. J Laryngol Otol 1985;99:793–794.

Hocutt JE, Corey GA, Rodney WM. Nasolaryngoscopy for family physicians. Am Fam Physician 1990;42:1257–1268.

Kaliner MA. Sinusitis update. Resp Digest 1993;2:7–8.

Lancer JM, Jones AS. Flexible fibreoptic rhinolaryngoscopy: results of 338 consecutive examinations. J Laryngol Otol 1985;99:771–773.

Lancer JM, Moir AA. The flexible fibreoptic rhinolaryngoscope. J Laryngol Otol 1985;99:767–770.

Patton D, DeWitt D. Flexible nasolaryngoscopy: a procedure for primary care. Prim Care Cancer 1992;12:13–21.

Rohr A, Hassner A, Saxon A. Rhinopharyngoscopy for the evaluation of allergic-immunologic disorders. Ann Allergy 1983;50(6):380–384.

Tenenbaum DJ. A buyer's guide to nasopharyngoscopes. Fam Pract Mgmt 1995;2:43–45.

CHAPTER 7

....

Simple Open Breast Biopsy

Open or surgical breast biopsy is performed for a wide variety of indications, although excluding the presence of breast cancer in a lump or lesion is the most common reason for performing the procedure. Open breast biopsy usually is performed only after radiologic (mammography or ultrasound) evaluation of both breasts. Fine-needle aspiration biopsy also may precede an open breast biopsy, adding additional support for the benign or low-risk nature of a lesion to be managed in the office setting.

Some physicians argue that breast surgeons are the only individuals who should perform an open breast biopsy. Many other surgical and medical specialists, however, can provide this service as part of quality care for the patient. The office setting is comfortable and familiar for most patients, and office biopsies can be performed at significant cost savings over similar procedures in other surgical settings.

There are specific indications when the family physician can provide this service safely and effectively (Table 7.1). Removal of symptomatic, persisting, benign-appearing, or low-risk lesions can be appropriately performed in the office setting. Women may remain anxious once a work-up has determined a lesion is benign, and may request removal by simple biopsy for peace of mind.

Lesions that are highly suspicious for malignancy, either because of cellular changes on fine-needle aspiration biopsy, characteristics at physical examination, or mammographic changes, may be appropriately referred to a breast surgeon for more definitive surgical intervention (Table 7.2). If it is likely that cancer is present, most surgeons prefer to perform the initial biopsy. More than 80% of the nearly 600,000 open breast biopsies performed every year in the United States are for benign disease, and many women can be selectively screened for office or hospital procedures.

Some have expressed concern regarding whether office biopsy is appropriate should an occult or unsuspected cancer be uncovered. Office biopsy does not interfere with cancer management; breast cancer is generally managed with two-stage procedures (biopsy followed by definitive surgery performed at a later date). Another historic barrier to office biopsy has been the recommendation that all specimens be examined by frozen section in order to perform hormone receptor assays. Hormone receptor evaluation now can be performed on specimens placed in formalin.

This chapter will focus on simple open biopsy techniques, and will not address the issues of nipple exploration for subareolar lesions, wide excision, needle localization biopsy, axillary node sampling, or flap creation associated with more extensive procedures on the breast.

METHODS AND MATERIALS

Patient Preparation

The patient is asked to undress from the waist up, given a gown, and laid in the supine position. The ipsilateral arm can be raised above the patient's head.

Nonsterile Tray for Anesthesia

Place the following items on a nonsterile sheet covering a Mayo stand:

   Nonsterile gloves

   Skin marking pen

   1 inch of 4×4 gauze

   Povidone-iodine solution placed on gauze

   10-mL syringe filled with 2% lidocaine with epinephrine (Xylocaine epinephrine)

   Short (¾ inch) 30-gauge needle and a long (1¼ inch) 27-gauge needle

Sterile Tray for the Procedure

Place the following items on a sterile drape covering the Mayo stand:

   Sterile gloves

   2 inches of sterile 4×4 gauze

   No. 15 scalpel and blade handle

TABLE 7.1.   Situations Appropriate for Simple Open Breast Biopsy

Low-risk	Persisting, symptomatic, or anxiety-producing lesions (negative mammogram, examination suggesting benign lesion, and negative needle aspiration biopsy)
Recurrent cysts that repeatedly refill following needle aspiration	To exclude a rare cystic carcinoma
Symptomatic fibroadenomas	In patients who request removal
Significant, persisting fibrocystic change	Producing excessive anxiety

TABLE 7.2. Situations Not Appropriate for Simple Open Breast Biopsy

Nonpalpable lesions noted on mammography	Perform stereotactic biopsy.
A mass deep in a large breast	Surgical removal may better be performed by an experienced physician in an operating room with general anesthesia.
Nipple discharge requiring meticulous duct dissection	Consider referral to a surgeon skilled in ductal surgery.
Lesion likely to be a breast cancer	Mammography, physical examination, and/or needle aspiration biopsy suggests the presence of malignancy. Consider referral to a surgeon for definitive care.

3 hemostats

Iris scissors

Allis tissue forceps

Metzenbaum (or other tissue-cutting) scissors

Needle holder

Adson forceps with teeth

Adson forceps without teeth

4-0 Vicryl suture (or other absorbable suture)

5-0 Prolene suture (or other nonabsorbable suture)

Disposable (nonsterile) battery cautery, inserted into a sterile glove

10-mL syringe, 18-gauge needle, and 27-gauge needle for additional anesthesia if needed

PROCEDURE DESCRIPTION

1. The patient is asked to undress from the waist up, given a gown, and laid in the supine position. The physician should identify the lesion and mark the skin over the mass in the event that the administration of the anesthetic obscures the margins. The skin incision is designed to maximize the cosmetic result (Fig. 7.1). A circumferential or semicircular incision usually is chosen, and can be hidden at the edge of the areola or beneath the breast if the lesion is in these locations. Alternately, a radial incision may be chosen for the inferior aspect of the breast.
2. Once the skin incision is drawn, the skin is anesthetized with 2% lidocaine with epinephrine. The skin is anesthetized using a 30-gauge needle, and then the subcutaneous fat (overlying the breast lesion) also is injected. A longer (1¼ inch) 27-gauge needle is substituted, and a field block is completed by administering anesthetic on all sides of the lesion.

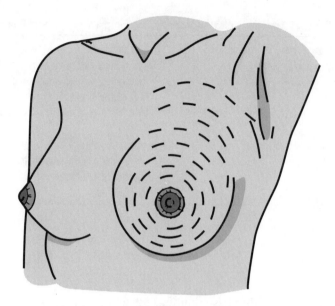

FIGURE 7.1. The skin incision should be a gentle curving arc over the lesion, following the skin lines of Langer. Alternatively, radial incisions may be made in the inferior aspect of the breast.

3. Skin incision is performed with a No. 15 scalpel blade held perpendicular to the skin surface. The incision is carried down to the subcutaneous fat. The lesion is palpated, and an incision is made around the lesion, attempting to remove a rim of normal tissue on all sides of the lesion. A hemostat or Allis tissue forceps (clamp) is used to grasp the lesion as it is being dissected from the surrounding breast tissue.

4. Traction can be applied with the Allis tissue forceps to raise the lesion, and to facilitate cutting beneath the lesion (Fig. 7.2). Repeated palpation is performed to ensure that the entire lesion is removed. Additional anesthetic may be required if the patient has discomfort during this part of the procedure, especially when cutting deep within the wound. Once the specimen is removed, the wound bed is palpated for a final time.

5. The anterior (skin) surface of the biopsy specimen can be marked with a nylon suture tag (Fig. 7.3). A Vicryl suture may be placed in the lesion to mark the 12 o'clock position (ends cut long) on the biopsy specimen, and dye or a second Vicryl suture is used to mark the 3 o'clock position (ends cut short). The lesion is placed in formalin and sent for histologic examination. Alternately, frozen sections can be performed, if desired and available. Hormone receptors now can be performed on lesions fixed in formalin, and are ordered only if the lesion should be malignant.

6. The breast is a highly vascular tissue that can bleed extensively at, or following, surgery. Hemostats can be placed on bleeding vessels, and battery electrocautery can be used to limit bleeding into the surgical field. Before wound closure is attempted, efforts should be made to stop all bleeding within the wound. 4-0 Vicryl suture could be placed in a "figure of 8" pattern to tie off the bleeding vessels.

7. Most experts discourage approximation of the defect deep in the breast tissue, because the resulting contour of the breast may be distorted by closing the dead space. Most authors no longer advocate drain placement. If the deep breast tissue is not closed, meticulous efforts at hemostasis should be undertaken to reduce the chances of a painful postoperative hematoma. A collection of fluid, or seroma, often develops in the breast tissue, which will slowly pull the breast tissue together as it resolves.

8. The skin and subcutaneous tissue can be closed with a running intracutaneous or subcutaneous closure (Fig. 7.4). 5-0 Vicryl suture can be used for subcutaneous closure, or alternately, an easy to pull-through 5-0 Prolene suture can be used for running intracuticular closure. Some authors recommend that interrupted nylon skin sutures should be avoided due to the cross hatching that is produced. Antibiotic cream can be placed

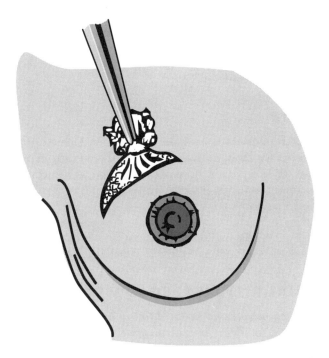

FIGURE 7.2.   The lesion is lifted with a clamp, completely excised, and the deep breast tissue is not sutured closed.

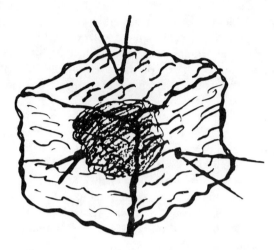

FIGURE 7.3. The specimen can be marked to orient the pathologist to the surfaces. A nylon suture can be placed on the anterior (top) surface, and Vicryl sutures placed in the lateral surfaces at 12 o'clock (long ends) and 3 o'clock (short ends).

over the wound to assist with skin healing. Adhesive tape (Steri-strips) is applied over the wound for additional strength.
9. Direct pressure is applied to the site for 10 minutes following the surgery. Gauze is placed over the wound site, and the patient should put on and wear a firm bra for additional support for the next 72 hours.

FOLLOW UP

* Most benign growths do not require any specific follow up. If a fibroadenoma or fibrocystic change is noted to be associated with atypical hyperplasia, the risk of subsequent development of breast cancer is increased. Patients demonstrating atypical hyperplasia at biopsy should receive frequent screening examinations.
* The discovery of malignancy or an in-situ cancer should prompt referral to a surgical oncologist for consideration of further intervention. Hormone receptor analysis should be performed if malignancy is discovered.

PROCEDURE PITFALLS/COMPLICATIONS

* ***The breast is bruised and painful following the procedure.*** Bruising is very common following breast surgery. Postoperative bruising can be reduced by efforts to control all bleeding points within the wound, and by applying pressure to the wound following the surgery. Painful hematomas can develop if the deep breast tissue is not sutured together, as

is currently recommended. Symptomatic, large hematomas may require needle drainage.

• *The wrong lesion was removed at biopsy.* When a lesion is not completely removed or the wrong lump is removed, a lawsuit may ensue. It is imperative that family physicians performing open breast biopsy have a high confidence level that the lesion in question can be readily identified. Lesions that cannot be palpated should be addressed with a different biopsy technique, such as stereotactic biopsy.

• *The breast has a crease and indentation following the procedure.* Some deformity and scarring is possible following any surgical breast procedure. No promises should be made to the patient regarding the final scar. Closing the deep breast defect created by the biopsy with an absorbable suture can produce an abnormal breast contour. Many experts advise leaving the deep space unsutured, allowing a seroma to form that will close the space over time. The subcutaneous tissue and skin are sutured closed.

• *It is difficult to mark the specimen for orientation before it is placed in formalin.* If an ellipse of skin is excised on top of the lesion, this can remain attached to the specimen and provide orientation to the anterior surface. If a standard incision is made, no skin is removed and

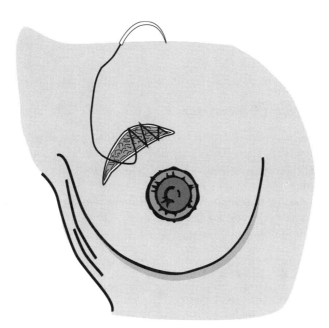

FIGURE 7.4.   The subcutaneous tissue and the skin are then sutured. The skin can be closed with subcutaneous 5-0 Vicryl suture.

the anterior surface should be marked. A nylon suture can be placed on the anterior surface to tag that site. A Vicryl suture can be placed in the lateral surfaces at 12 o'clock and 3 o'clock to mark those sites. Alternately, dye can be painted onto one of the surfaces. The pathology slip should indicate which marking system is used.

- *Colleagues argue that office biopsy should only be performed when frozen sections can be done to evaluate the need for hormone receptor determination.* A historic barrier to office biopsy was the inability to perform hormone receptor evaluation on specimens placed in formalin; however, performing all low-risk breast biopsies in medical centers with immediate frozen section availability is expensive and uses extensive medical services. Newer pathology techniques allow hormone receptor analysis on office specimens placed in formalin. Check with the pathologist to determine how best to handle the tissue.

TABLE 7.3. CPT Codes

CPT Code	Description	1998 Total RVUs[a]	1998 Average 50% Fees in U.S.[b]
19101	Incisional biopsy	7	$548
19120	Excision lesion(s)	9.06	$698

CPT only © 1998 American Medical Association. All rights reserved.

[a] Department of Health and Human Services, Health Care Financing Administration. Medicare program: revisions to payment policies and adjustments to the relative value units (RVUs) under the physician fee schedule for calendar year 1998. Federal Register 42 CFR part 414. October 31, 1997; 62(211):59103–59255.

[b] 1998 Physicians' Fee Reference. West Allis, WI: Yale Wasserman, DMD, Medical Publishers, 1998.

PHYSICIAN TRAINING

Physicians performing open breast biopsy should possess general surgical and suturing skills. These skills may be obtained during residency training. Physicians should be prepared to control brisk intraoperative bleeding. While the technique for simple open breast biopsy is fairly basic, 10 to 20 precepted procedures may be needed before a physician is comfortable performing the procedure unassisted. The greatest skill may be the selection of appropriate candidates for simple open biopsy.

ORDERING INFORMATION

Fine-tipped battery surgical cautery (General Medical Corporation, 8741 Landmark Road, Richmond, VA 23228; 804-264-7500)

Allis tissue forceps (7¼ inch, 5×6 teeth, straight), Metzenbaum scissors (7 inch, curved, standard), Iris scissors (4 inch, straight, standard pattern)

(Miltex Surgical Instruments, 6 Ohio Drive—CB5006, Lake Success, NY 11042; 800-645-8000)

Vicryl (polyglactin) and nylon sutures (Ethicon, P.O. Box 151, Sommerville, NJ 08876; 908-218-0707)

BIBLIOGRAPHY

Bellantone R, Rossi S, Lombardi CP, Cinini C, Minelli S, Cracitti F. Excisional breast biopsy: when, why, and how? Int Surg 1995;80:75-78.

DeWitt DE. Office procedures: a step-by-step guide to open breast biopsy. Consultant 1994;34:1151-1164.

Donegan WL. Evaluation of a palpable breast mass. N Engl J Med 1992;327:937-942.

Economou SG, Economou TS. Atlas of surgical techniques. Philadelphia: WB Saunders, 1996:99-119.

Fisher ER, Sass R, Fisher B. Biologic considerations regarding the one and two step procedures in the management of patients with invasive carcinoma of the breast. Surg Gynecol Obstet 1985;161:245-249.

Foster RS. Biopsy techniques. In: Harris JR, Lippmman ME, Morrow M, Hellman S, eds. Diseases of the breast. Philadelphia: Lippincott-Raven, 1996:133-138.

Giuliano AE. Breast. In: Way LW, ed. Current surgical diagnosis and treatment. 10th ed. Norwalk, CT: Lange, 1994:293-316.

Isaacs JH. Breast biopsy and the surgical treatment of early carcinoma of the breast. Obstet Gynecol Clin North Am 1987;14:711-732.

Painter RW, Clark WE, Deckers PJ. Negative findings on fine-needle aspiration biopsy of solid breast masses: patient management. Am J Surg 1988;155:387-390.

Shumate CR. Surgical evaluation and treatment of breast cancer. In: Blackwell RE, Grotting JC, eds. Diagnosis and management of breast disease. Cambridge, MA: Blackwell Science, 1996:211-224.

CHAPTER 8

Punch Biopsy of the Skin

Skin biopsy is the most important diagnostic test for skin disorders. In selected patients, a properly performed skin biopsy almost always yields useful diagnostic information. Some authors believe that most errors in dermatologic diagnosis occur because of failure to perform a prompt skin biopsy.

Punch biopsy is considered the primary technique to obtain diagnostic full-thickness skin specimens. It is performed using a circular blade or trephine attached to a pencil-like handle. The instrument is rotated down through the epidermis, dermis, and into the subcutaneous fat. The punch biopsy yields a cylindrical core of tissue that must be gently handled (usually with a needle) to prevent crush artifact at the pathologic evaluation.

Punch biopsy sites can be closed with a single suture, and generally produce only a minimal scar. Since linear closure is performed on the circular defect, stretching the skin before the punch biopsy allows the relaxed skin defect to appear more elliptical, and makes it easier to close. The skin is stretched perpendicular to the relaxed skin tension lines, so that the resulting ellipse and closure is parallel to these skin tension lines.

Punch biopsy of inflammatory dermatoses can provide useful information when the differential diagnosis has been narrowed. Cutaneous neoplasms can be evaluated by punch biopsy, and the discovery of malignancy may alter the planned surgical excision procedure. Routine biopsy of skin rashes is not recommended, because the commonly reported nonspecific pathology result rarely alters clinical management.

METHODS AND MATERIALS

Equipment

Nonsterile Tray for Anesthesia

Place the following items on a nonsterile sheet covering a Mayo stand:

Nonsterile gloves

1 inch of 4×4 gauze soaked with povidone-iodine solution

3-mL syringe filled with 2% lidocaine with epinephrine (Xylocaine with epinephrine), and a 30-gauge needle

Labeled formalin container(s) for the number of biopsies to be performed

Sterile Tray for the Procedure

Place the following items on a sterile sheet covering a Mayo stand:

Sterile gloves (Some physicians choose to perform the procedure using the nonsterile gloves used for anesthesia.)

Desired punch biopsy instrument (3 or 4 mm)

Needle holder for suturing

Desired size suture (4-0, 5-0, or 6-0 nylon suture, depending upon body site)

Iris scissors

21-gauge, 1¼-inch needle for elevating the specimen, if a sterile instrument is used (alternately, the nonsterile anesthesia needle can be used)

Sterile fenestrated drape (some physicians choose to perform the procedure without a covering drape)

PROCEDURE DESCRIPTION

1. The area to be biopsied should be selected. Commonly selected sites are the most abnormal-appearing site within a lesion or the edge of an actively growing lesion.
2. The skin is cleansed with povidone-iodine solution, and anesthetized with 2% lidocaine with epinephrine. A 30-gauge needle is used for administering an anesthetic to limit discomfort.
3. The lines of least skin tension should be identified for the area to be biopsied. For example, on the arm, these lines run perpendicular to the long axis of the extremity. The incision line created by the suturing after the biopsy will be oriented parallel to the lines of least skin tension. Physicians who cannot recall the line orientation for a specific body area should consult the widely published drawings of these lines.
4. The skin surrounding the biopsy site is stretched with the thumb and index finger of the nondominant hand (Fig. 8.1). The skin is stretched perpendicular to the lines of least skin tension. When the skin relaxes after the circular biopsy is performed, an elliptical-shaped wound exists that is oriented in the same direction as the lines of least skin tension. On the arm, the skin is stretched along the long axis of the extremity.
5. The punch biopsy instrument is held vertically over the skin and rotated downward using a twirling motion created by the first two fingers on the dominant hand (Fig. 8.2). Once the punch instrument has penetrated beneath the dermis into the fat, or once the instrument reaches the hub, it is removed.
6. The cylindrical skin specimen is elevated with the anesthesia needle held in the nondominant hand. The use of forceps is discouraged, as these

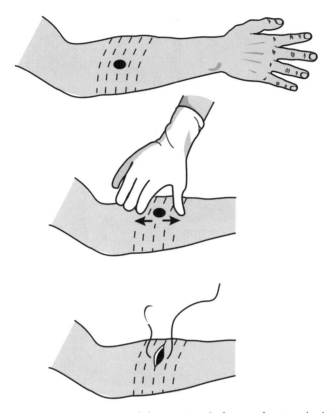

FIGURE 8.1. Orienting a punch biopsy. Just before performing the biopsy, the lines of least skin tension are determined. The skin is stretched 90 degrees (perpendicular) to the lines of least skin tension using the nondominant hand, and the punch biopsy is performed. Following relaxation of the distending hand, the skin appears as an elliptical effect that can be closed with sutures parallel to the lines of least skin tension.

instruments frequently cause crush artifact. Scissors held in the dominant hand cut the specimen free from the subcutaneous tissues. Make the cut below the level of the dermis.

7. The wound is closed with one or two interrupted nylon sutures. 5-0 nylon is used for most nonfacial areas, and 6-0 nylon is used for most facial wounds. The suture generally creates good hemostasis, and antibiotic ointment and a bandage are then applied.

FOLLOW UP

- *Melanoma.* A punch biopsy revealing malignancy usually mandates further surgical intervention. If the lesion is a thin melanoma (less than 0.75-mm

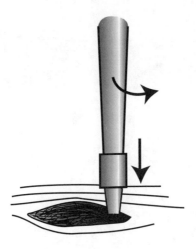

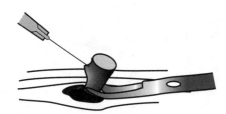

FIGURE 8.2.   Punch biopsy technique. The punch biopsy instrument is held perpendicular to the surface of the lesion. The instrument is pressed down into the lesion while it is rotated clockwise and counterclockwise, cutting down to the subcutaneous fat. The punch biopsy instrument is removed, and the biopsy specimen is gently lifted to avoid crush artifact. Scissors are used to cut the specimen free at a level below the skin. Small punch biopsy defects do not require suturing, while larger wounds (4 or 5 mm) should be closed to reduce healing time and scarring.

thick), and the specimen was from an area of average thickness for the lesion, then the family physician can perform the excision of the lesion with at least a 5-mm margin of normal surrounding skin. If the lesion is a thicker melanoma, consider a referral to a melanoma center for excision and sentinel node removal following dye injection.
• *Other Skin Malignancy.* Basal cell carcinoma and squamous cell carcinoma can be completely excised with a 4- to 6-mm margin of normal appearing

skin. The larger margin (6 mm) is recommended for larger tumors, recurring tumors, or tumors on high-risk sites such as the nose, ears, and eyelids. Other, less common tumors, such as dermatosarcoma protuberans, may require referral for more extensive surgical management.

- *Benign Growths.* The follow-up of benign growths depends on the particular lesion, patient preference, and cosmetic concerns. Some patients may prefer to leave a benign growth alone. Others may request a fusiform excision or shave excision. Some benign growths that are premalignant (such as actinic keratoses) can be managed with ablative cryotherapy, or peeled off with 5-fluorouracil therapy.
- *Inflammatory Lesions.* The specific cause for an inflammatory skin change should be sought. Further medical testing (e.g., x-rays or blood work) that can be ordered depends on the information provided in the report from the pathologist. For example, an angiotensin-converting enzyme level might be ordered if the skin biopsy reveals sarcoidosis. Sometimes the pathologist cannot define the specific inflammatory lesion, but can narrow the differential diagnosis for the clinician to allow for therapeutic intervention.
- *Chronic Skin Disorders.* Chronic papulosquamous disorders or other skin problems can be correctly identified, and proper therapy initiated. An example is a patient with an early psoriasis plaque, whose atypical-appearing lesion was correctly identified by punch biopsy.

TABLE 8.1. CPT Codes

CPT Codes	Description	Total 1998 RVUs[a]	1998 Average 50% Fees in U.S.[b]
11100	Skin biopsy—one lesion [separate procedure]	1.36	$110
11101	Biopsy—each separate/additional lesion [separate procedure]	0.72	$74

CPT only © 1998 American Medical Association. All rights reserved.

[a] Department of Health and Human Services, Health Care Financing Administration. Medicare program: revisions to payment policies and 5-year review of and adjustments to the relative value units (RVUs) under the physician fee schedule for calendar year 1998. Federal Register 42 CFR part 414. October 31, 1997; 62(211):59103–59255.

[b] 1998 Physicians' Fee Reference. West Allis, WI: Yale Wasserman, DMD, Medical Publishers, 1998.

PROCEDURE PITFALLS/COMPLICATIONS

- *The procedure is uncomfortable for the patient.* This procedure should rarely be associated with discomfort. Slow and adequate anesthesia infiltration of the area should make this a painless procedure. If the anesthetic is administered subcutaneously rather than intradermally, it may take a minute for full anesthetic effect, compared to the almost immediate effect of intradermal administration.

- *Nerve injury develops from the procedure.* Many physicians have been taught to rotate the punch instrument down to the hub. This produces a circular incision that may penetrate up to ⅜ inch below the skin surface, depending upon which punch instrument is used. On the areas where the skin is thin, such as the face or dorsum of the hand, it is possible to damage arteries, nerves, and veins below the skin. Most physicians can identify when the instrument penetrates through the skin, because a "give" can be felt. Once the instrument has penetrated the dermis into the subcutaneous fat, cease downward pressure. Use care when punch biopsy procedures are performed on the face, neck, or distal extremities.

- *It is time consuming to switch from nonsterile to sterile gloves.* Many physicians perform the procedure using the nonsterile gloves used for anesthesia. While this means that the suturing is performed with nonsterile gloves, it is very unusual for infection to develop at a punch biopsy site.

PHYSICIAN TRAINING

Punch biopsy is a simple technique to learn and perform. Supervision is rarely needed after a physician has performed two or three procedures. General surgical and suture-tying skills are needed when suture closure of the wound is routinely performed.

ORDERING INFORMATION

Punch biopsy instruments (Fray Products Corporation, Baird Research Park, 1576 Sweet Home Road, Amherst, NY 14228; marketed through Delasco, 608 13th Avenue, Council Bluffs, IA 51501, 800-831-6273.)

BIBLIOGRAPHY

Brown JS. Minor surgery: a text and atlas. 3rd ed. New York: Chapman & Hall, 1997.

Fewkes JL. Skin biopsy: the four types and how best to perform them. Prim Care Cancer 1993;13:35-39.

Pariser RJ. Skin biopsy: lesion selection and optimal technique. Modern Med 1989;57:82-90.

Paver RD. Practical procedures in dermatology. Austr Fam Physician 1990; 19:699-701.

Phillips PK, Pariser DM, Pariser RJ. Cosmetic procedures we all perform. Cutis 1994;53:187-191.

Stegman SJ. Basics of dermatologic surgery. Chicago: Year Book Medical Publishers, 1982.

Swanson NA. Atlas of cutaneous surgery. Boston: Little Brown, 1987.

Wheeland RG, ed. Cutaneous surgery. Philadelphia: WB Saunders, 1994.

Zuber TJ. Skin biopsy techniques: when and how to perform punch biopsy. Consultant 1994;34:1467-1470.

THERAPEUTIC PROCEDURES

CHAPTER 9

··

Bartholin's Cyst/Abscess Marsupialization

The Bartholin's glands are two small lubricating glands located at the base of the labia minora. The glands provide lubrication to the vulvar and vaginal tissues, but are not essential for vaginal lubrication during sexual intercourse. The ducts draining the glands open mucosally near the entrance to the vagina. When the ducts draining the Bartholin's glands become obstructed, the glands can become enlarged and cystic, or become infected and abscessed. Most often the duct obstruction results from nonspecific inflammation or trauma to the tissues.

Bartholin's cysts may vary from 1 to 8 cm in diameter, and most are asymptomatic; however, cysts may become symptomatic at any size, and can then be considered for treatment. Abscesses usually develop rapidly, and produce acute pain and difficulty with walking or sitting. Once infection develops, the tissues usually appear erythematous, swollen, and may exhibit localized hemorrhage. Many abscesses rupture spontaneously after 4 days, but women usually request intervention before then.

Marsupialization involves removal of the roof of the Bartholin's gland and suturing the walls of the gland directly to the skin above. Recurrence rates for abscesses are reduced with this technique, but, occasionally, excessive scarring can be seen. Electrocautery may be needed during the procedure to control bleeding from the skin, especially when the procedure is performed on inflamed glands. Many authorities consider marsupialization to be the treatment of choice for Bartholin's cysts and abscesses.

Many authorities believe that asymptomatic cysts in women younger than 40 years of age do not require surgical intervention. Some have advocated the total excision of cysts in women older than age 45 because of the association with adenocarcinoma. At least one recent review does not advocate this intervention because of the rarity of the cancer.

ALTERNATE PROCEDURES

Marsupialization has advantages over the alternative procedures for treating Bartholin's cysts and abscesses. Simple incision and drainage provides adequate symptom relief of enlarged or abscessed Bartholin's glands, but this procedure has a high recurrence rate. A small, balloon-tipped (Word) catheter can be placed inside the gland and left in place for 4 to 6 weeks, creating a chronic fistula tract to help reduce recurrence. Although the technique is easy to perform, some patients find avoiding sexual intercourse and having the foreign body in place for such a long period unacceptable. Another option is the complete excision of the enlarged gland. This, however, is a complex procedure that can have significant bleeding complications.

DIFFERENTIAL DIAGNOSES

Mesonephric cysts of the vagina (usually more proximal in the vagina than Bartholin's cysts)

Epithelial inclusion cysts (usually more superficial than Bartholin's cysts)

Lipoma or fibroma (usually more firm than Bartholin's cysts)

Sebaceous cyst and abscess of the skin (yellow, sebaceous material inside may help identify these lesions)

Varicosities (bluish color may help to identify its vascular nature)

Perianal abscesses extending anteriorly (usually tenderness extends back towards the anus)

METHODS AND MATERIALS

Patient Preparation

The patient undresses from the waist down and puts on a gown. An absorbent sheet is placed beneath the patient. The patient can be left seated on the table, to speak with the physician before the procedure. The patient is then placed in the lithotomy position for the procedure.

Equipment

Nonsterile Tray for Anesthesia

Place the following items on a nonsterile tray:

Nonsterile gloves

4×4 gauze

Povidone-iodine solution

2 10-mL syringes with 27-gauge 1¼-inch needles filled with 2% lidocaine with epinephrine (Xylocaine with epinephrine)

Mask

Place the following items on a sterile drape covering the Mayo stand:

Sterile gloves

3 hemostats (Mosquito clamps)

No. 15 blade and blade handle (No. 11 blade can be used alternately)

Needle holder

3-0 Vicryl suture

2 inches of 4×4 gauze

Mayo or tissue scissors

Iris scissors (for cutting sutures)

Adson forceps with teeth

2 Allis forceps for holding tissue edges

Sterile battery electrocautery (can reuse the disposable units if the tip is cleaned and disinfected in glutaraldehyde [Cidex], and the unit is slipped inside a sterile glove that is on the surgery tray, and only the tip is allowed to protrude through the tip of one of the fingers of the glove)

Procedure Description

1. The patient is placed in the lithotomy position. The labial area is cleansed with povidone-iodine solution. A fenestrated drape can be placed to cover the area.
2. The skin above and surrounding the cyst on all sides is anesthetized with 2% lidocaine with epinephrine. Two 10-mL syringes may be required to produce adequate anesthesia.
3. It helps to have a gloved assistant retract the labia majora laterally. The operator can place a gloved finger inside the vagina to stabilize the cyst and move it forward to the introitus.
4. A vertical fusiform skin incision (about 1 inch long and ½ inch wide) is made at the mucocutaneous junction over the top of the cyst using a No. 15 blade (Fig. 9.1A). The incision should not extend onto the vaginal verge, perineal tissues, or toward the anus. If tissue inflammation is present, excessive bleeding may be noted and electrocautery may be needed. The incision is then extended deeper into the cyst (be prepared for splatter), and the roof of the cyst is removed using scissors or a scalpel blade.
5. The cyst contents should be removed and cultured, if desired, and the cyst cavity irrigated. Culturing cysts is unlikely to provide useful information, while culturing abscesses can guide antibiotic therapy. Septae pres-

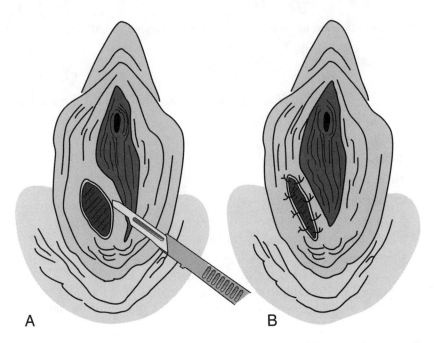

A   B

FIGURE 9.1. **A.** The cyst roof is excised with No. 15 blade. **B.** The cyst wall is sutured to the overlying skin with Vicryl sutures.

ent within the cavity may need to be broken up with a finger or instrument. Palpate the cyst wall for nodular or irregular areas that could suggest the presence of malignancy. If any areas of concern are found, especially in older women, consider performing an excisional biopsy of the abnormal area.

6. The edges of the cyst wall are grasped and pinched upward next to the vaginal mucosa. Interrupted, absorbable sutures, such as 3-0 Vicryl, can be used to approximate the cyst wall to the overlying skin and mucosa (Fig. 9.1B). Usually seven to 14 sutures are needed, depending on the wound size.

7. Iodoform gauze can be used to pack the wound, especially if the cavity is deep. Shallow or smaller wounds can be managed with topical antibiotic cream and dry gauze applied to cover the wound. Some physicians choose to examine the wound in 3 to 7 days to make sure that the wound edges are not growing together, causing the cyst to reform.

FOLLOW UP

- Pathology reports are not usually generated unless total excision or a localized biopsy is performed. If the report suggests a coexisting adenocarcinoma, refer the patient to a gynecologic oncologist.

- Physicians may request culture and sensitivity reports on the cyst contents. Testing for gonorrhea may be appropriate, depending on the patient's age and risk factors. Because of the high rate of sterile cysts, the benefit of routinely culturing all cysts is debatable; however, culturing abscesses may guide antibiotic selection and may be useful.

- Recurrent cysts are a difficult problem, and many family physicians will consider referring the patient to a gynecologist if a recurrence develops after the initial treatment. Fortunately, recurrences are less likely following marsupialization.

PROCEDURE PITFALLS/COMPLICATIONS

- *Arterial bleeding.* Arterial bleeding can develop after any surgical procedure involving Bartholin's cysts or abscesses. Puncturing an artery is more likely if the initial incision is made through the vulvar skin, rather than through the vaginal mucosa. Arterial bleeding also may accompany excision procedures, or if the posterior wall of the cyst is excised or curetted. Late bleeding may also occur after the patient goes home, when the spasm in a cut arteriole is relieved and the vessel reopens.

- *Recurrence of cysts/abscesses after the procedure.* Recurrence can follow any procedure, but is most likely after simple incision and drainage. Some physicians follow up 1 week after marsupialization to ensure that the wound edges do not grow together and the cyst does not reform.

- *Sepsis after surgery on an abscess.* The medical literature reports rare occurrences of systemic infection after surgical intervention. One recent report described septic shock complicating abscess drainage. If there is evidence of cellulitis or infection, coverage for gram-positive, gram-negative and anaerobic bacteria is recommended.

- *Bleeding from the skin at the surgical procedure.* When inflammation is present in the tissues, any incision can produce extensive bleeding. Hospitalization and transfusions are occasionally required for extensive bleeding. It is recommended that electrocautery be available for Bartholin's procedures, either sterile battery or sterile electrosurgical cautery.

- *Excessive vulvar scarring after marsupialization procedures.* Incisions made through the vulvar skin can produce excessive scarring, which may remain tender for years. Incisions made through the vaginal mucosa can reduce the incidence of this complication.

TABLE 9.1.   CPT Codes

CPT Codes	Description	1998 Total RVUs[a]	1998 Average 50% Fees in U.S.[b]
56420	Incision and drainage of Bartholin's gland abscess	2.32	$175
56440	Marsupialization of Bartholin's gland cyst	5.99	$578
56740	Excision of Bartholin's gland or cyst	7.18	$698
56605	Biopsy vulva; one lesion [separate procedure]	1.93	$170

CPT only © 1998 American Medical Association. All rights reserved.
[a] Department of Health and Human Services, Health Care Financing Administration. Medicare program: revisions to payment policies and adjustments to the relative value units (RVUs) under the physician fee schedule for calendar year 1998. Federal Register 42 CFR part 414. October 31, 1997; 62(211):59103–59255.
[b] 1998 Physicians' Fee Reference. West Allis, WI: Yale Wasserman, DMD, Medical Publishers, 1998.

PHYSICIAN TRAINING

Marsupialization of a Bartholin's cyst requires good general surgical skills. Physicians with extensive training and experience in general and skin surgery can become proficient in the technique after several precepted procedures. Physicians with less surgical training in their residency should perform many supervised procedures before attempting this procedure alone. The complication rates of Bartholin's cyst procedures should be respected, and patients can be referred to more experienced physicians if the family physician lacks adequate experience.

ORDERING INFORMATION

All materials can be obtained from listings in other chapters.

BIBLIOGRAPHY

Andersen PG, Christensen S, Detlefsen GU, Kem-Hansen P. Treatment of Bartholin's abscess: marsupialization versus incision, curettage, and suture under antibiotic cover. A randomized study with 6 months' follow up. Acta Obstet Gynecol Scand 1992;71:59-62.

Cunha B. Bartholin's gland abscess. Emerg Med 1994;26:85-86.

Droegemueller W, Herbst AL, Mishell DR, Stenchever MA. Comprehensive gynecology. St Louis: CV Mosby, 1987:569-571.

Graber RF. Marsupialization of a Bartholin's gland cyst. Patient Care 1987;21:135-136.

Greenhill JP, Corson SL, Sedlacek TV, Hoffman JJ. Greenhill's surgical gynecology. 5th ed. Chicago: Year Book Medical Publishers, 1986:58-63.

Heah J. Method of treatment for cysts and abscesses of Bartholin's gland [Editorial]. Br J Obstet Gynecol 1988;95:321-322.

Hoosen AA, Nteta C, Moodley J, Sturm AW. Sexually transmitted diseases including HIV infection in women with Bartholin's gland abscess. Genitourin Med 1995;71:155-157.

Lopez-Zeno JA, Ross E, O'Grady JP. Septic shock complicating drainage of a Bartholin gland abscess. Obstet Gynecol 1990;76:915-916.

Visco AG, Del Priore G. Postmenopausal Bartholin gland enlargement: a hospital-based cancer risk assessment. Obstet Gynecol 1996;87:286-290.

Word B. New instrument for office treatment of cyst and abscess of Bartholin's gland. JAMA 1964;190:167-8.

CHAPTER 10

Eyelid Chalazia

Chalazia are chronic inflammatory granulomas of the meibomian glands of the eyelid. These are the most common type of eyelid masses.

The meibomian glands are long, sebaceous glands within the tarsal plate. Chalazia may develop either on the conjunctival or the external skin side of the eyelid. These granulomas usually contain a gelatinous material, surrounded by an inflammatory reaction. Chalazia are more common on the upper lid, and are associated with seborrheic dermatitis, chronic blepharitis, and rosacea.

Chalazia follow a variable course. Many chalazia undergo spontaneous resorption; therefore, observing the lesions for a few months is a very reasonable management plan. Chalazia may erode through to the skin or conjunctival surfaces, with drainage of the gelatinous contents. Chronic or persisting chalazia are generally treated surgically, most often because of patient discomfort, eye irritation, or cosmetic concerns.

The incision and curettage removal technique is preferred because of its simplicity and good outcomes. This technique is easy to learn, and office removal is much cheaper for patients than similar surgical procedures in other settings (e.g., surgicenters or outpatient surgical suites).

ALTERNATIVE PROCEDURES

Triamcinolone acetonide (Kenalog) (0.1 to 0.3 mL) injected into the lesion. Results appear comparable with either the 10 or 40 mg/mL concentration. Complications of the steroid injections include skin atrophy, skin depigmentation, and central retinal artery occlusion.

Excision of chalazia. The entire sac can be lifted out from the surrounding tissues and excised with scissors or electrosurgical loop excision. This procedure causes more tissue defect than incision and curettage. If this tissue defect is on the conjunctival surface, the patient may feel it during the first few postoperative days.

Ablation of the granuloma with electrocautery, chemicals, cryosurgery, or laser. Ablation procedures have the potential for excessive scar reactions, which, in essence, replaces the previous chalazion mass. Use of cautery or chemicals deep within the tissue can produce tattooing or dimpling.

METHODS AND MATERIALS

Patient Preparation

The patient is placed in a supine position, with an absorbent sheet draped inside the patient's collar and over the upper chest. Place several tissues in the patient's hand.

Equipment

Place the following items on a drape covering the Mayo stand:

Nonsterile gloves

Mask

3-mL syringe filled with 2% lidocaine with epinephrine (Xylocaine with epinephrine); 30-gauge needle

Fine-tipped Adson forceps without teeth

Iris scissors

Sterile 2-mm chalazion curette and sterile 3-mm chalazion curette (remove whichever curette is desired from its sterile pouch at the time of the procedure)

1 chalazion clamp

Sterile No. 11 blade

1 inch of 4×4 gauze

Refrigerated bottle of proparacaine hydrochloride 0.5% ophthalmic solution (Ophthetic)

1 bottle of saline eye wash

Tobramycin (Tobrex) ophthalmic ointment

6 small, cotton-tipped applicators

Gentamicin sulfate (Garamycin) or ciprofloxacin hydrochloride (Ciloxan) ophthalmic solution

1 adult eye shield with a small swirl of tobramycin ointment inside the shield

Suction cup applicator for the eye shield

PROCEDURE DESCRIPTION

1. Patient is placed in a supine position with the head firmly supported.
2. Proparacaine hydrochloride 0.5% ophthalmic solution is liberally administered to the patient's affected eye. The solution initially produces some burning.
3. A plastic eye shield containing a thin film of tobramycin ophthalmic ointment on the inside of it is gently placed over the globe. The suction

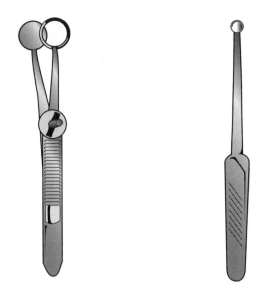

FIGURE 10.1. Chalazion forceps (clamp) and curette.

cup is attached to the convex (outer) portion of the shield for insertion and removal. The shield is gently slid under the upper eyelid as the patient looks down. The patient then looks up, the lower lid is pulled down, and the shield is slid beneath the lower eyelid.

4. Additional proparacaine hydrochloride 0.5% anesthetic can be applied at this time.

5. 2% lidocaine with epinephrine (Xylocaine) is injected adjacent to the chalazion, using a 30-gauge needle. The anesthetic is administered through the conjunctival surface if the chalazion is pointing inward, or through the skin if the chalazion is pointing outward. The needle must always point away from the globe.

6. The chalazion clamp can be applied now, if used (Fig. 10.1). The flat portion of the clamp is placed against the skin, and the chalazion should protrude through the open ring. The clamp screw is lightly tightened. Bleeding can be effectively controlled during the procedure with the clamp. If the clamp is not used, bleeding can be controlled by applying pressure with the fingers of the nondominant hand.

7. An incision is made into the chalazion with a No. 11 blade. Orient the incision vertically (perpendicular to the eyelid margin) if it is made through the conjunctiva, and horizontally (parallel to the eyelid margin) at least 3 mm from the edge if it is made through the external skin of the eyelid.

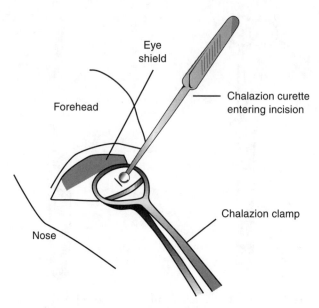

FIGURE 10.2.   Chalazion curette entering incision.

8. A 2- or 3-mm chalazion curette is placed within the chalazion (Fig. 10.2). The gelatinous material is extruded and wiped onto gauze. A cotton-tipped swab can be used to press around the chalazion and help extrude the material.
9. The walls of the chalazion are scraped vigorously with the curette to scar it down and reduce the chance of recurrence.
10. Bleeding can usually be controlled with the application of direct pressure using gauze. Some physicians prefer to use electrocautery inside the defect to control bleeding and induce scarring.
11. The clamp is removed. The shield is removed. Any blood that remains inside the lids can be washed out using proparacaine hydrochloride 0.5% or an eye irrigation solution. A few drops of an antibiotic solution (gentamicin sulfate or ciprofloxacin hydrochloride ophthalmic) are applied. The patient holds gauze gently over the eyelid for 5 to 10 minutes before leaving the office. The nurse or assistant ensures that adequate hemostasis exists, and gives the patient the postprocedure handout. The patient should be reassured that some blurring of vision frequently follows use of the eye shield.

FOLLOW UP

• Pathology reports are not usually generated from this procedure unless a total excision is performed. If excision is needed for a lesion that is not cystic, the possibility of a rare malignancy must be excluded. Ophthalmology referral should be considered for unusual or atypical lesions.

• Culture and sensitivity testing generally are not necessary for chronic lesions. *Staphylococci* or *streptococci* can be cultured from an acute hordeolum, but chalazia are commonly sterile cysts.

• Recurrent cysts are a difficult problem, and many primary physicians will refer patients to an ophthalmologist if lesions recur frequently.

• Some physicians choose to reexamine the eyelid in 3 to 4 weeks to check for lesion recurrence or the development of nearby lesions.

PROCEDURE PITFALLS/COMPLICATIONS

• *The patient complains of discomfort when the eye shield is applied.* Adequate topical anesthetic should be administered before application of the eyeshield. Warn the patient when applying proparacaine hydrochloride 0.5% that the solution is cold and may cause burning. Allow the patient to have a sense of control by blotting away excess solution with some hand-held tissues. When the eye shield is ready to be placed, lubricate the inside (concave) surface with a small amount of tobramycin ophthalmic ointment. The eye shield should be manipulated by applying the suction cup to the convex surface. Gently slip in the shield as detailed in the procedure description. If a chalazion clamp is used, be sure it is not pressing the eye shield into the eyeball.

• *The patient moves suddenly during the injection of local anesthetic.* The needle tip should always be directed away from the globe, even if the eye shield is in place. The patient should always be warned of the impending needle-stick, and strongly urged to hold still. Local anesthetic administration with a 30-gauge needle at a very slow rate can improve patient cooperation during the procedure.

• *The chalazion curette punctures through the opposite side of the eyelid.* Care must be used when scraping with the curette. The flat (underside) of the chalazion clamp can reduce this complication, but appropriate caution should be exercised.

• *Other tumors of the eyelids can masquerade as chalazia.* If an eyelid tumor does not behave like a normal chalazia, does not yield gelatinous material or recurs, consider an excisional biopsy of the lesion for histologic confirmation.

• *Silver nitrate cautery to the walls of the chalazia can produce tattooing.* Silver nitrate is best used for superficial application, not deep within soft tissues. The silver salts can stain the tissues and leave a permanent discoloration. Silver nitrate cautery is not advocated for chalazion removal.

• *Patients may complain of recurrence.* Chalazia frequently recur, but there also may be multiple chalazia within one eyelid. One chalazion may be excised, only to leave an adjacent one, to the dismay of the patient. Always palpate the lid after chalazion removal to ensure successful eradication of the diseased tissue.

TABLE 10.1.   CPT Codes for Chalazion Removal

CPT Codes	Description	1998 Total RVUs[a]	1998 Average 50% Fees in U.S.[b]
67800	Chalazion excision—one	2.37	$150
67801	Multiple chalazia—same lid	3.35	$215
67805	Multiple chalazia—different lids	3.68	$255

CPT only © 1998 American Medical Association. All rights reserved.

[a] Department of Health and Human Services, Health Care Financing Administration. Medicare program: revisions to payment policies and adjustments to the relative value units (RVUs) under the physician fee schedule for calendar year 1998. Federal Register 42 CFR part 414. October 31, 1997;62(211);59103–59255.

[b] 1998 Physicians' Fee Reference. West Allis, WI: Yale Wasserman, DMD, Medical Publishers, 1998.

PHYSICIAN TRAINING

Chalazion removal is best learned by direct, hands-on experience. The technique is simple, and once a physician has gained familiarity with the instruments, he or she may feel comfortable performing the procedure without supervision after four to five supervised procedures.

ORDERING INFORMATION

Ciprofloxacin hydrochloride 3.5 mg/mL ophthalmic solution (2.5-mL bottle; Ciloxan, Alcon Laboratories, 6201 South Freeway, Fort Worth, TX 76134; 817-293-0450, or through a local pharmacy)

Corneal eye shields, large (blue) and medium (green) (Ellman International, 1135 Railroad Avenue, Hewlett, NY 11557; 800-835-5355)

Gentamicin sulfate 3 mg/mL ophthalmic solution (5-mL bottle; Garamycin, Schering-Plough, 2000 Galloping Hill Road, Kenilworth, NJ 07003; 908-298-4000, or through a local pharmacy)

Hunt chalazion forceps (clamp), 4 inches long, inside ring diameter 12 mm (Miltex Instrument Company, 6 Ohio Drive, Lake Success, NY 11042; 800-645-8000)

Meyhoefer chalazion curettes, 5 inches long, size 2 (2 mm) and size 4 (3.5 mm) (Miltex Instrument Company, 6 Ohio Drive, Lake Success, NY 11042; 800-645-8000)

Proparacaine hydrochloride 0.5% ophthalmic solution (15-mL bottle, refrigerated; Alcaine, Alcon Laboratories, 6201 South Freeway, Fort Worth, TX 76134; 817-293-0450, or through a local pharmacy)

Surgitron electrosurgical unit with fine-point cautery tip (Ellman International, 1135 Railroad Avenue, Hewlett, NY 11557; 800-835-5355)

Tobramycin 0.3% ophthalmic ointment (3.5-g tube; Tobrex, Alcon Laboratories, 6201 South Freeway, Fort Worth, TX 76134; 817-293-0450, or through a local pharmacy)

BIBLIOGRAPHY

Black RL, Terry JE. Treatment of chalazia with intralesional triamcinolone injection. J Am Optom Assoc 1990;61:904–906.

Cottrell DG, Bosanquet RC, Fawcett IM. Chalazions: the frequency of spontaneous resolution [Letter]. Br Med J (Clin Res Ed) 1983;287:1595.

Diegel JT. Eyelid problems. Blepharitis, hordeola, and chalazia. Postgrad Med 1986; 80:271–272.

Diegel JT. Surgery for chalazion. In: Benjamin RB, ed. Atlas of outpatient and office surgery. 2nd ed. Philadelphia: Lea & Febiger, 1994:22–25.

Epstein GA, Putterman AM. Combined excision and drainage with intralesional corticosteroid injection in the treatment of chronic chalazia. Arch Ophthalmol 1988;106:514–516.

Garrett GW, Gillespie ME, Mannix BC. Adrenocorticosteroid injection vs. conservative therapy in the treatment of chalazia. Ann Ophthalmol 1988;20:196–198.

MacRae DW. Tumors and related lesions of the eyelids and conjunctiva. In: Peyman GA, Sanders DR, Goldberg MF, eds. Principles and practice of ophthalmology. Philadelphia: WB Saunders, 1980:2218–2243.

Procope JA, Kidwell EDR. Delayed postoperative hemorrhage complicating chalazion surgery. J Natl Med Assoc 1994;86:865–866.

Vidaurri LJ, Pe'er J. Intralesional corticosteroid treatment of chalazia. Ann Ophthalmol 1986;18:339–340.

CHAPTER 11

···

Minimal Excision Technique for Epidermoid (Sebaceous) Cysts

Epidermoid cysts are asymptomatic, slowly enlarging, firm to fluctuant, dome-shaped lesions that frequently appear on the trunk, neck, face, or scrotum, or behind the ears. Occasionally, a dark keratin plug (a comedo) can be seen overlying the cyst cavity. These epithelial, walled cysts vary in size from a few millimeters up to 5 cm. The cysts are mobile within the skin, unless fibrosis exists from a previous inflammation.

The term sebaceous cyst has fallen into disuse; other terms used now include epidermal cyst, keratin cyst, epithelial cyst, and epidermoid cyst. Other types of cysts are included in Table 11.1. These cysts often arise from a ruptured pilosebaceous follicle associated with acne. Duct obstruction of a sebaceous gland in the hair follicle can result in a long, narrow channel opening in the surface comedo. Other causes include a developmental defect of the sebaceous duct or traumatic implantation of surface epithelium beneath the skin.

The cysts contain keratin and lipid, and the rancid odor often associated with these lesions relates to the relative content of fat, presence of bacterial infection, or decomposition. Spontaneous rupture of the cysts discharges the soft, yellow, keratin material into the dermis. A tremendous inflammatory response (foreign body reaction) ensues, often producing a sterile purulent material. Scarring of these inflamed cysts makes removal more difficult.

Most cysts are simple lesions, but a few special situations should be considered. Multiple epidermoid cysts (associated with lipomas or fibromas of the skin) and osteomas should be considered as part of Gardner's syndrome with associated premalignant colonic polyps. Dermoid cysts of the head often can be confused with epidermoid cysts, and attempted removal of a dermoid cyst can create a wound with intracranial communication. Some cysts can be associated with basal cell and squamous cell carcinoma, and some authors advocate histologic evaluation of the wall of all removed cysts. The rarity of associated cancer makes histologic evaluation necessary only when solid tumors or unusual findings are present.

97

TABLE 11.1. Major Lesions in the Differential Diagnosis

Pilar cysts	Lipomas	Steatocystomas
Milia	Dermoid cysts	Fibrous tissue tumors
Myxoid cysts	Median raphe cysts	Thyroglossal duct cysts
Parotid tumors	Gardner's syndrome	Preauricular cyst
Pilonidal cyst	Branchial cleft cyst	Favre-Racouchot syndrome

Cyst infection can develop spontaneously or following rupture. It is often unclear whether an inflamed cyst is infected, and many physicians prefer to treat these lesions with antibiotics, incision, and drainage. Excision and closure can be very difficult with inflamed cysts, and it may be preferable to postpone a surgical procedure until the inflammation has subsided (typically 1 week).

There are many surgical approaches to epidermoid cysts. While complete surgical excision can ensure removal of the sac and prevent recurrence, this technique is time-consuming and requires suture closure. The minimal excisional technique has been proposed as a less invasive, but successful, intervention. The minimal excision uses a 2- to 3-mm incision, expression of the cyst contents, and extraction of the cyst wall through the incision. Vigorous finger compression is used to express the cyst contents and loosens the cyst wall from surrounding tissues to facilitate removal of the sac. The tiny wound can be closed with a single suture, although most physicians do not close this opening. A variation of this technique uses a punch biopsy instrument to create the opening into the cyst.

Expression of the cyst contents through the small opening can cause the sebaceous material to spray across the surgery room. Gauze can be used to cover the area as compression is applied, or a clear, adhesive splatter control shield can be used to cover the site. Some practices require protective eye wear for the procedure.

Simple incision and drainage of cysts frequently results in recurrence. Two iodine crystals can be placed into the center of the cyst, and over the next few weeks the cyst becomes dark brown and hard. This hard nodule can then be expressed from the skin. This simple technique is inexpensive, but the need for a follow up and the length of time for lesion removal may make this technique less desirable to many patients.

OTHER TYPES OF EPITHELIAL CYSTS

* Pilar or trichilemmal cyst (wen). These cysts occur predominantly on the scalp, are odorless, and have less fat and more keratin than epidermoid cysts. These are very amenable to removal by the minimal excision technique.

- Dermoid cyst. These congenital cysts occur in the lines of cleavage, and occur sublingually around the eyes and on the base of the nose. These cysts have a rancid odor. The lesions can extend intracranially, and preoperative computed tomographic (CT) scanning is recommended.
- Milia. These 1- to 2-mm lesions can arise spontaneously or due to trauma. A small nick in the epidermis with a No. 11 blade allows expression of the keratinaceous white kernel.
- Steatocystoma multiplex. These multiple, small, yellow, cystic nodules (a few millimeters in size) can be found on the trunk, upper arms, axilla, and thighs. The multitude of lesions may preclude removal of all of the cysts.
- Favre-Racouchot syndrome. These multiple lesions on the face result from profound sun damage. The pilosebaceous openings stretch and the orifices fill with keratin material, producing comedones and cysts.

METHODS AND MATERIALS

Equipment

Nonsterile Tray for Anesthesia

Place the following items on a nonfenestrated sheet covering a Mayo stand:

Nonsterile gloves and mask

1 inch of 4×4 gauze soaked with povidone-iodine solution

1 inch of 4×4 gauze

1 5-mL syringe, filled with 2% lidocaine with epinephrine (Xylocaine with epinephrine), with a 30-gauge needle attached

25-gauge, 1¼-inch needle (for anesthetizing beneath the cyst)

Sterile Tray for the Procedure

Place the following items on a sterile disposable sheet covering a Mayo stand:

Sterile gloves

Fenestrated disposable drape

2 sterile bandages to anchor the drape

3 small-tipped hemostats (Mosquito clamps)

No. 11 blade

Needle holder for suturing (if needed)

Iris scissors

Adson forceps

2 inches of 4×4 sterile gauze

Suture materials (if needed)

Splatter control shield (if desired)

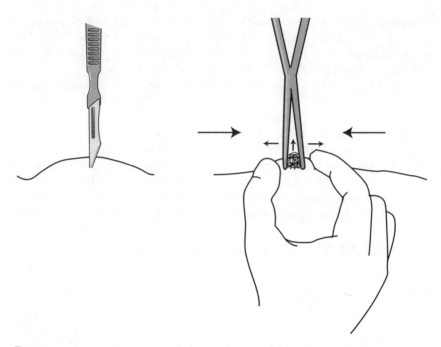

FIGURE 11.1. Incision is made into the top of the cyst using a No. 11 blade. The cyst is squeezed to remove all of the cyst contents. A hemostat can be placed into the incision, and the blades opened while the cyst is squeezed, to facilitate removal of the cyst contents.

Some physicians will use the nonsterile gloves used for administering the anesthesia for the removal of small or superficial cysts.

PROCEDURE DESCRIPTION

1. The skin overlying the site is cleansed with povidone-iodine solution. The skin overlying the cyst and the tissue to the sides and beneath the cyst are anesthetized with 2% lidocaine with epinephrine.
2. A fenestrated drape can be placed on the patient, with the lesion beneath the fenestration. A No. 11 blade is used to create a stab incision into the center of the cyst. A small-tipped hemostat is placed into the cyst, the tips gently opened, and compression applied to allow the cyst contents to pass through the opening (Fig. 11.1).
3. The hemostat can be removed, and both thumbs are used to express the cyst contents. Gauze or a splatter shield can be used to shield the physician

from splatter. The hemostat can be reinserted, if needed, to assist with passage of the sebaceous material.

4. Following vigorous and complete expression, the hemostat is reintroduced into the cyst cavity and the capsule at the base of the wound is grasped and elevated. Attempt to gently remove the entire sac through the small opening (Fig. 11.2). The sac may break, and several pieces may need to be removed.

5. At the end of the procedure, the wound should be inspected to ensure that all of the cyst wall has been removed. The sac wall can be pieced together to provide additional confirmation of complete removal.

6. Direct pressure is applied to the site with gauze. Antibiotic ointment and gauze is taped over the site. The patient is encouraged to hold direct pressure (using gauze) to the site for 1 to 2 hours following the procedure. Most small incisions do not require suture closure.

FOLLOW UP

Malignant growths may require a second procedure to provide a wider margin of excision around the original lesion. Malignancy may rarely be detected at the original surgery. Once the cyst contents have been squeezed out, a mass may be palpated adjacent to the cyst, suggesting that a tumor may be present. It is recommended that the minimal technique be abandoned for a formal excision if a solid tumor is detected. If malignancy is discovered in a cyst wall that is removed at the time of the minimal surgical technique, consider a second excision.

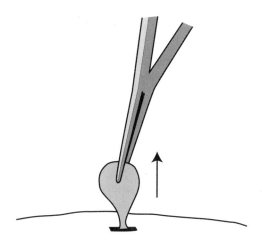

FIGURE 11.2. After vigorous squeezing, removing the cyst contents, and loosening the cyst wall from the surrounding tissue, a hemostat is placed in the wound and the entire cyst wall is gently delivered through the small incision.

TABLE 11.2. CPT Codes: Excision of Benign Lesions

CPT Codes[a]	Description	1998 Total RVUs[b]	1998 Average 50% Fees in U.S.[c]
11400	Trunk, arms, legs 0.5 cm or less	1.49	$124
11401	Trunk, arms, legs 0.6 to 1.0 cm	2.05	$150
11402	Trunk, arms, legs 1.1 to 2.0 cm	2.59	$200
11403	Trunk, arms, legs 2.1 to 3.0 cm	3.22	$264
11404	Trunk, arms, legs 3.1 to 4.0 cm	3.75	$353
11406	Trunk, arms, legs over 4.0 cm	4.97	$452
11420	Scalp, neck, hand, foot, genitalia 0.5 cm or less	1.63	$138
11421	Scalp, neck, hand, foot, genitalia 0.6 to 1.0 cm	2.31	$164
11422	Scalp, neck, hand, foot, genitalia 1.1 to 2.0 cm	2.80	$223
11423	Scalp, neck, hand, foot, genitalia 2.1 to 3.0 cm	3.63	$317
11424	Scalp, neck, hand, foot, genitalia 3.1 to 4.0 cm	4.17	$395
11426	Scalp, neck, hand, foot, genitalia over 4.0 cm	5.90	$504
11440	Face, ear, eyelid, nose, lip, mm 0.5 cm or less	1.90	$150
11441	Face, ear, eyelid, nose, lip, mm 0.6 to 1.0 cm	2.54	$197
11442	Face, ear, eyelid, nose, lip, mm 1.1 to 2.0 cm	3.10	$265
11443	Face, ear, eyelid, nose, lip, mm 2.1 to 3.0 cm	4.09	$355
11444	Face, ear, eyelid, nose, lip, mm 3.1 to 4.0 cm	5.03	$475
11446	Face, ear, eyelid, nose, lip, mm over 4.0	6.45	$594

mm, mucous membranes.

CPT only © 1998 American Medical Association. All rights reserved.

[a] If malignancy is associated with the lesion, then the malignant excision codes (11600–11646) can be reported.
[b] Department of Health and Human Services, Health Care Financing Administration. Medicare program: revisions to payment policies and adjustments to the relative value units (RVUs) under the physician fee schedule for calendar year 1998. Federal Register 42 CFR part 414. October 31, 1997;62(211):59103–59255.
[c] 1998 Physicians' Fee Reference. West Allis, WI: Yale Wasserman, DMD, Medical Publishers, 1998.

Because malignancy is so rarely associated with cancer, some physicians feel it is not cost-effective to send all epidermoid cyst walls for histologic evaluation. Others feel that all specimens should be sent because cancer has been noted in the literature. Certainly any atypical-appearing lesion or one associated with a palpable irregularity in the cyst wall should be sent to the pathologist for analysis.

Many lesions can be confused with epidermoid cysts. If a solid tumor is discovered at the time of the procedure, a biopsy should be obtained. Incisional biopsy can be performed for very large lesions, and excisional biopsy for the smaller lesions. Pilar tumors of the scalp are often confused with epidermoid cysts, and may require wide excision as they can erode into the skull.

Simple epidermoid cysts that appear to be completely excised do not generally require a follow-up visit. If a recurrence is brought to the physician's attention at a later date, standard surgical excision should be attempted.

PROCEDURE PITFALLS/COMPLICATIONS

- *The contents of the cyst sprayed.* Vigorous expression of the cyst contents can cause material to literally fly across the room. Gauze should be loosely held over the site to prevent spraying. Masks and eye protection may be needed for the physicians, and care should be used to avoid spraying the nursing personnel. Some physicians use a splatter control shield to avoid this problem.

- *The cyst wall will not come out of the tiny incision.* Cysts that have previously ruptured or been inflamed may have significant adjacent scarring. The scarring may preclude removal with the minimal excision technique. In addition, less-experienced physicians are often not vigorous enough when compressing the cyst. Pressure applied with the thumbs can loosen the cyst wall from the surrounding tissues. Inability to remove the cyst should result in a formal excision procedure.

- *The cyst wall breaks during the procedure.* Cyst wall breakage during the procedure may relate to the surgical technique or the anatomic location of the cyst. Cysts on the scalp (trichilemmal cysts or wens) may have thicker walls than typical epidermoid cysts on the face. Many physicians report that it is easier to remove scalp cysts intact. Thin-walled cysts tend to break, and may need to be removed in pieces; however, if adequate kneading of the skin occurs before attempted removal, many of the cysts can be removed intact.

- *A blood clot developed after cyst wall removal.* Removal of large cysts can create a significant open space beneath the skin. Hematomas or infections can fill this space. Major bleeding is rarely associated with this procedure, and hematomas can be avoided by applying 1 to 2 hours of firm pressure (using gauze) to the surgical site. Direct pressure can also express any clot that may develop at this site.

- *Expressing the cyst contents is tiring.* The minimal excision technique can be physically demanding when performed correctly. Despite the amount of work that is required, this technique can be very gratifying to both physician and patient. Using the thumbs to express the cyst contents achieves greater pressure.

- *Cyst contents could not be expressed.* Solid tumors may masquerade as a typical epidermoid cyst. The pilar cyst or pilar tumor of the scalp can be confused with a typical cyst, and the pilar tumor can invade surrounding tissues. If a solid tumor is suspected during minimal excision, the area should be removed for histologic examination by a formal surgical excision.

PHYSICIAN TRAINING

Formal training is needed for the techniques of anesthetic administration, lesion excision, and closure if it is performed. Most family physicians receive the necessary surgical skills during their residency training. Others could obtain this training with the assistance of an experienced preceptor. Most physicians experienced in skin surgery can perform these procedures unsupervised after three to five procedures.

ORDERING INFORMATION

Taut splatter control shield (adherent, see-through plastic bag that prevents material spraying from the cyst; approximately $2.50 per shield) (Taut Inc., 2571 Kaneville Court, Geneva, IL 60134; 630-232-8005, 800-231-8288)

BIBLIOGRAPHY

Avakoff JC. Microincision for removing sebaceous cysts [Letter]. Plast Reconstr Surg 1989;84:173–174.

Cruz AB, Aust JB. Lesions of the skin and subcutaneous tissue. In: Hardy JD, Kukora JS, Pass HI, eds. Hardy's textbook of surgery. Philadelphia: JB Lippincott, 1983:319–328.

Domonkos AN, Arnold HL, Odom RB. Andrews' diseases of the skin: clinical dermatology. 7th ed. Philadelphia: WB Saunders, 1982.

Foroughi D, Britton P. When is a "wen" a "wen"?: a diagnostic dilemma. Br J Plastic Surg 1984;37:379–382.

Habif TP. Clinical dermatology. 2nd ed. St Louis: Mosby, 1990.

Humeniuk HM, Lask GP. Treatment of benign cutaneous lesions. In: Parish LC, Lask GP, eds. Aesthetic dermatology. New York: McGraw-Hill, 1991:39–49.

Johnson RA. Cyst removal: punch, push, pull. Skin 1995;1:14-15.

Klin B, Ashkenazi H. Sebaceous cyst excision with minimal surgery. Am Fam Physician 1990;41:1746-1748.

Morgan RF, Dellon AL, Hoopes JE. Pilar tumors. Plast Reconstr Surg 1979;63:520-524.

Parlette HL. Management of cutaneous cysts. In: Wheeland RG, ed. Cutaneous surgery. Philadelphia: WB Saunders, 1994:647-663.

Vogt HB, Nelson RE. Excision of sebaceous cysts: a nontraditional method. Postgrad Med 1986;80:128-134.

C H A P T E R   12

Hemorrhoidectomy for Thrombosed External Hemorrhoids

External hemorrhoids usually develop over time, and may result from straining with stools, childbirth, lengthy car trips or prolonged sitting, constipation, or diarrhea. External hemorrhoids represent distended vascular tissue in the anal canal distal (outside) to the dentate line (the junction between the rectal mucosa and the specialized skin of the anal canal, called the anoderm). External hemorrhoids are covered by anoderm and perianal skin that are richly innervated with somatic pain fibers. Diseases affecting the anal canal or the external hemorrhoidal vessels can be very painful.

External hemorrhoids often develop in healthy young individuals, and may suddenly become thrombosed. Thrombosed external hemorrhoids usually present with pain with standing, sitting, or defecation. The thrombosis is slowly absorbed by the body over the course of several weeks. A resolving thrombosis may erode through the skin and produce bleeding or drainage.

Acutely swollen and tender thrombosed external hemorrhoids can be surgically removed if the physician encounters them in the first 72 hours after onset. After 72 hours, the discomfort of the procedure often exceeds the relief provided by the surgery. Some patients still may chose to undergo late surgery, although they need to understand that without surgery the hemorrhoid will eventually become fibrosed and resolve over days to weeks.

An elliptical incision can be made over the thrombosis, and the clot and the entire diseased hemorrhoidal plexus can be removed in one piece. Although the site can be left open, many physicians prefer to place subcutaneous sutures to limit postoperative pain and bleeding. Suturing in this area, historically, has been avoided because of fear of complications, yet the rich vascular network in the anal tissues usually provides for rapid healing.

Simple incision over a thrombus after the administration of local anesthesia can be performed to remove the clot, but this procedure has been associated with a significant rate of rethrombosis. Many experts now recommend excision of the entire thrombosis and external hemorrhoidal vessels beneath. This procedure is more extensive than simple incision, but usually yields better outcomes.

METHODS AND MATERIALS

Patient Preparation

The patient should get undressed from the waist down and should be draped. An absorbent pad is placed beneath the patient. The patient can be seated to speak with the physician. At the start of the procedure, the patient is rolled to the left side in the left lateral decubitus position. The right hip and knee are flexed, and a sheet covers the patient's legs.

Equipment

Nonsterile Tray for Anoscopy and Anesthesia

Place the following items on a nonsterile drape covering the Mayo stand:

Nonsterile gloves

1 inch of 4×4 gauze

Povidone-iodine solution (on 4×4 gauze)

1 inch of 2% lidocaine jelly (Xylocaine) (placed on the corner of the drape)

Ives anoscope

Mask (if desired)

10-mL syringe filled with 1% lidocaine with a 25-gauge 1¼-inch needle attached

Sterile Tray for the Procedure

Place the following items on a sterile drape covering the Mayo stand:

Sterile gloves

2 inches of sterile 4×4 gauze

3 hemostats (Mosquito clamps)

No. 15 scalpel blade and blade handle

Needle holder

Adson forceps with teeth

Iris scissors (for cutting sutures)

Mayo or tissue cutting scissors

Allis clamp for holding tissue

4-0 Vicryl suture

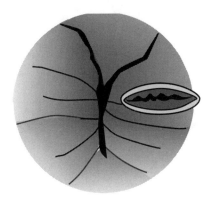 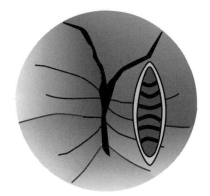

Radial incision   Circumferential incision

FIGURE 12.1. The circumferential incision of a thrombosed external hemorrhoid opens across the hemorrhoidal plexus, making removal of clots from the vessel easier.

PROCEDURE DESCRIPTION

1. The patient is placed in the left lateral decubitus position. The perianal skin is visualized by having an assistant separate the buttocks or by taping the buttocks apart. The anal canal can be visualized using an Ives anoscope coated with 2% lidocaine jelly. The extent of the hemorrhoidal disease should be assessed and coexisting anal pathology excluded before initiating the procedure. Alternately, anoscopy can be performed after anesthetic administration (injection) when the thrombosed hemorrhoids are exquisitely tender.

2. The perianal skin and anal canal are cleansed with povidone-iodine solution. The base of the hemorrhoid is infiltrated with at least 5 mL of 1% lidocaine, using a 25-gauge 1¼-inch needle. Avoid making multiple needle sticks in the anal tissues because the puncture sites can bleed after needle removal. Warn the patient about impending needle insertion into the tender tissues.

3. A fusiform (elliptical) excision is made into the anal skin overlying the thrombosis. It is preferable to make a radial incision extending out from the anal canal if the entire hemorrhoid plexus is removed, other physicians prefer a circumferential incision that exposes more clots by crossing over more of the hemorrhoidal sinusoids beneath (Fig. 12.1). Vigorous bleeding may accompany this incision, and can be controlled with direct pressure or electrocautery, if needed.

4. A clamp can be placed on the fusiform skin island and traction applied to the skin to reveal the hemorrhoid below (Fig. 12.2). The entire hemorrhoid is sharply excised with a No. 15 blade or scissors. The entire

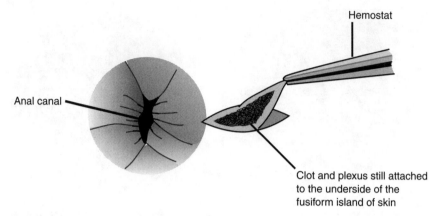

FIGURE 12.2.   The fusiform island of skin is grasped and elevated. Sharp dissection is performed of the clot and hemorrhoidal plexus of vessels in the subcutaneous tissues.

hemorrhoidal plexus usually can be removed as one piece attached to the fusiform skin island. Avoid cutting into the muscle sphincter below the hemorrhoidal vessels.

5. Once the hemorrhoidal plexus and clot have been removed, the base of the wound is examined for residual small clots. Additional hemorrhoidal tissue or clots can be sharply excised. Some physicians chose to close the deep wound with subcutaneous, absorbable, buried 4-0 Vicryl sutures to avoid significant postprocedure bleeding. The sutures should be completely subcutaneous and not penetrate external to the anal skin. Wound closure can reduce bleeding and discomfort from the surgical site. Alternately, some physicians prefer to leave the wound open.

6. The wound should be inspected for adequate hemostasis. If epinephrine is used to anesthetize the wound and the wound is unsutured, late bleeding (up to several hours after the procedure) can develop once the epinephrine wears off. Topical antibiotic ointment is applied to the surgical site, and 1 inch of 4×4 gauze is applied over the site between the buttocks. The patient can be given additional gauze for replacement at home.

FOLLOW UP

• Most physicians believe that the thrombosed plexus of vessels should not be sent to the pathologist, as analysis of the tissue generally fails to yield useful additional information. If solid tumors or unusual tissue characteristics are discovered at the time of surgery, histologic analysis of the tissue may be warranted.

- The patient should have a follow-up visit at 6 weeks. If extensive coexistent internal hemorrhoids are noted, these can be managed with infrared coagulation or other destructive modalities. Some physicians also recommend colon examination for all patients with hemorrhoids. The medical literature provides conflicting recommendations on the need for colon evaluation, but if flexible sigmoidoscopy is performed, it should be done 6 to 12 weeks after the original surgery.

PROCEDURE PITFALLS/COMPLICATIONS

- *The patient left the office with the wound dry, but returned later with extensive bleeding.* Hemorrhoidal plexuses include both arterial and venous vessels. When surgery is performed, the cut arterioles may spasm and bleeding ceases. If the surgical wound is not closed with sutures, the patient can develop significant bleeding. This scenario occurs more often when lidocaine with epinephrine is used for anesthesia. Some physicians advocate no epinephrine in the anesthetic and wound closure to limit the risk of late bleeding.

- *Excessive scarring or anal stenosis developed after the surgery.* The development of anal stenosis is a rare, but definite, complication associated with hemorrhoid surgery. The complication can be reduced by avoiding circumferential procedures on all sides of the anal canal. Performing extensive cautery can limit bleeding during the procedure, but also can induce extensive scarring and should be avoided.

- *Concern about risk of infection if wound is closed surgically.* Infection after suture closure is an unusual occurrence, partly because of the rich vascular network in the anal area. Several studies have confirmed the safety of suture closure, and discomfort and bleeding complications may be reduced by this technique. Antibiotics are used by some physicians for infection prophylaxis after suture closure.

- *Patient complains that anoscopy is too uncomfortable to perform before hemorrhoid surgery.* Extensive inspection of the perianal tissues is recommended to exclude coexisting disease. Infectious complications of the excision procedure may relate to unrecognized infectious processes, such as perianal abscesses. Persisting pain could relate to a coexisting fissure. The inspection of the anal tissues should not be deferred, and anoscopy can be performed after administration of the anesthetic to make it more tolerable for the patient.

- *Subcuticular wound closure is very difficult at the anus.* Suture placement is difficult in the anus because of the narrow surgical field, and because sutures do not hold well in the tissues below the anoderm. Taking adequate bites of tissue with each pass of the suture needle, and placing multiple, interrupted, buried sutures can ensure proper closure of the wound. The suture should be subcuticular and not protrude through the anoderm.

- *The patient notices a tearing sensation and bleeding in the first week after the procedure.* Passage of hard stool can easily tear the suture line after the procedure. The need for soft stools must be emphasized to the patient. Multiple modalities can be used to soften the stools, such as stool softeners, stool-bulking agents, and increased daily consumption of fluids. Even with soft stools, however, it is not unusual for some tearing to occur at the suture line.

TABLE 12.1.   CPT Codes

CPT Codes[a]	Description	1998 Total RVUs[b]	1998 Average 50% Fee in U.S.[c]
46083	Incision of thrombosed hemorrhoid; external	2.11	$149
46250	Complete external hemorrhoidectomy	7.89	$714
46320	Enucleation/excision of external thrombosed hemorrhoid	2.42	$174

[a] The code selection depends on the procedure performed. If the complete hemorrhoidectomy is performed, as described in this chapter, then code 46250 can be reported.
CPT only © 1998 American Medical Association. All rights reserved.
[b] Department of Health and Human Services, Health Care Financing Administration. Medicare program: revisions to payment policies and adjustments to the relative value units (RVUs) under the physician fee schedule for calendar year 1998. Federal Register 42 CFR part 414. October 31, 1997;62(211):59103–59255.
[c] 1998 Physicians' Fee Reference. West Allis, WI: Yale Wasserman, DMD, Medical Publishers, 1998.

PHYSICIAN TRAINING

Physicians with proper surgical skills can master this procedure. Extensive training and experience in general and skin surgery may be needed before attempting this procedure unsupervised. The bleeding that occurs during the procedure may scare novice surgeons. The complications of the procedure should be respected, and patients can be referred to more experienced physicians if the family physician lacks a comfort level and adequate experience; however, the basic skills needed to perform this procedure are not unlike the fusiform excisional biopsy commonly performed for removal of skin lesions.

ORDERING INFORMATION

Instruments (hemostats, needle holder, blade handle, Iris scissors, Adson forceps, Allis clamps, Mayo scissors) (Miltex Instrument Company, 6 Ohio Drive, Lake Success, NY 11042; 800-645-8000)

Ives anoscope (Redfield Corporation, 210 Summit Avenue, Montvale, NJ 07645; 800-678-4472)

Lidocaine hydrochloride 2% jelly (Xylocaine jelly, Astra Pharmaceuticals, 50 Otis Street, Westborough, MA 01581; 508-366-1100)

BIBLIOGRAPHY

Bassford T. Treatment of common anorectal disorders [Review]. Am Fam Physician 1992;45(4):1787–1794.

Buls JG. Excision of thrombosed external hemorrhoids. Hosp Med 1994;30:39–42.

Ferguson EF. Alternatives in the treatment of hemorrhoidal disease. S Med J 1988;81:606–610.

Fry RD, Kodner IJ. Anorectal disorders. Clin Symposia 1985;37:10.

Gehringer GR, Levin IA. Office management of hemorrhoids. Female Patient 1982;7:21–26.

Grosz CR. A surgical treatment of thrombosed external hemorrhoids. Dis Colon Rectum 1990;33(3):249–250.

Leibach JR, Cerda JJ. Hemorrhoids: modern treatment methods. Hosp Med 1991;27:53–68.

Muldoon JP. The completely closed hemorrhoidectomy: a reliable and trusted friend for 25 years. Dis Colon Rectum 1981;24(3):211–214.

Schussman LC, Lutz LJ. Outpatient management of hemorrhoids. Prim Care 1986;13(3):527–541.

Zuber TJ. Anorectal disease and hemorrhoids. In: Taylor RB, ed. Manual of family practice. Boston: Little Brown, 1997:381–384.

CHAPTER 13

···

Infrared Coagulation of Internal Hemorrhoids

Infrared coagulation (IRC) is a safe, effective office therapy for first-, second-, and third-degree internal hemorrhoids. A 0.7-cm light tip transmits the infrared energy to the superior aspect of the hemorrhoid. A 1.25- to 1.5-second pulse of energy is applied, limiting the depth of tissue destruction. The treatment is well tolerated by the patient, and produces an eschar that tethers the hemorrhoid to the underlying tissue. Three to five exposures to each hemorrhoid generally reduce the blood flow and shrink the hemorrhoid.

The anal cushions are blood-filled sacs that reduce the effects of stool passing through the anal canal. Over time, the chronic passage of hard stool or straining can cause the anal cushions to lose the internal fibrous tissue support. The cushions then dilate with blood and prolapse into the anal canal, thus becoming hemorrhoids.

Internal hemorrhoids occur above the dentate line, at the junction between the rectal mucosa and the specialized anoderm of the anal canal. The rectal mucosa is generally not innervated above the dentate line, and internal hemorrhoids generally do not produce pain. The major symptoms produced by internal hemorrhoids are bleeding, protrusion, sensation of a lump, or bright red blood on the toilet tissue.

In general, the patient is examined while lying in the left lateral decubitus position (left side down on the table), with the physician on the side of the examination table (patient's head to the left, feet to the right) facing the patient's back. Internal hemorrhoids frequently occur in three consistent locations within the anal canal. The three locations are the right posterior position (10 o'clock), the right anterior position (2 o'clock), and the left lateral position (6 o'clock). All three positions should be thoroughly inspected before therapy is initiated.

Internal hemorrhoids are graded from 1 to 4. First-degree internal hemorrhoids do not protrude from the anus, and only extend into the lumen of the anal canal. Second-degree internal hemorrhoids protrude through the anus, usually with defecation, but spontaneously reduce. Third-degree internal hemorrhoids protrude and must be manually reduced. Fourth-degree

115

internal hemorrhoids protrude continuously and cannot be manually reduced. Family physicians most frequently encounter first- and second-degree internal hemorrhoids.

Many operative and nonoperative treatment options exist for symptomatic internal hemorrhoids. Rubber band ligation is a commonly performed intervention with high success rates. Recent reports of complications, such as pelvic sepsis, massive bleeding, pelvic thrombophlebitis, and death, have made this therapeutic option less popular. IRC has become the nonoperative treatment of choice in many family practice offices.

METHODS AND MATERIALS

Patient Preparation

The patient should be asked to undress from the waist down. A drape is placed over the legs and abdomen. An absorbent pad should be placed beneath the patient's buttocks. The patient can be left sitting to speak with the physician. The patient will be placed in the left lateral decubitus position with the left leg extended and the right (upper) leg slightly flexed at the hip and knee for the procedure.

Equipment

Place the following items on a nonsterile drape covering the Mayo stand:

  2 pairs of nonsterile gloves

  2 inches of 4 × 4 gauze

  3 large cotton-tipped swabs

  Ives anoscope

  1 inch of water soluble lubricating jelly (K-Y)

  1 inch of 5% lidocaine ointment (Xylocaine)

  Infrared coagulator assembled, plugged into the wall outlet, with the timer set at 1.25 seconds

PROCEDURE DESCRIPTION

1. The patient is placed in the left lateral decubitus position, with the right leg flexed over the extended left leg. Rectal examination is performed with the gloved index finger, checking the prostate (male patients) and examining for pathology, and lubricating the canal with 5% lidocaine ointment.
2. The lubricating jelly is applied to the Ives anoscope. The anoscope is

inserted three times, examining the right posterior, right anterior, and left lateral hemorrhoidal plexuses. The presence and severity of hemorrhoidal tissue is noted, using a light (flexible halogen lamp) to visualize inside the anoscope.

3. Once the anal tissues have been evaluated and the presence of disease noted, the Ives anoscope is reinserted, exposing the hemorrhoidal plexus to be treated. A large cotton-tipped swab is used to remove any stool that may be overlying the hemorrhoid. The examiner's nondominant hand should maintain the position of the anoscope.

4. The infrared coagulator handpiece is held in the dominant hand. The instrument is activated once outside of the patient to ensure proper functioning. The tip of the instrument is positioned against the upper portion of the hemorrhoid. The tip should be placed on the mucosal surface without deeply compressing the hemorrhoid.

5. The patient is warned of possible discomfort from the treatment before the infrared coagulator is activated to allow the patient to prepare. Several treatments can be administered in an arc pattern to the top (proximal portion) of the hemorrhoid (Fig. 13.1). The tip can be wiped clean with moist gauze after each infrared coagulator activation.

6. Alternately, a diamond pattern to the coagulator applications can be performed (Fig. 13.1). Warn the patient about applications performed near the dentate line, because increased sensation at this location may cause the patient to experience more discomfort at this site compared with applications to the upper (proximal) hemorrhoid.

7. Stop the procedure if the patient cannot tolerate the treatment, or if the patient needs a break. Usually four to six nonoverlapping applications are adequate to treat most hemorrhoid pads. Avoid treating all three

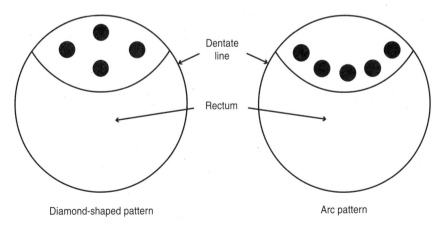

Diamond-shaped pattern   Arc pattern

FIGURE 13.1.   Infrared coagulation treatment patterns.

pads in one setting; the rare development of anal stenosis can follow circumferential treatment.

8. The anal tissues are wiped clear of all lubricating jelly once the procedure is completed. The patient is gradually and slowly brought to a standing position, watching for dizziness. Encouraging the patient to walk after the procedure can reduce some of the perceived discomfort from the treatment.

FOLLOW UP

- Many physicians chose to perform flexible sigmoidoscopy 6 weeks after infrared treatment to examine for coexisting colon pathology. The medical literature contains conflicting recommendations on colon evaluation of all patients presenting with hemorrhoids. This follow-up visit, however, can serve as an opportunity to reexamine the anal canal. If additional treatments are required, they can be performed at that visit; however, the CPT code for destruction of internal hemorrhoids carries a 90-day (3-month) global surgical period. Many insurance companies, including Medicare, refuse to reimburse for any additional treatments until 3 months after the initial treatment.
- Patients may have bloody drainage with their stools in the first few weeks after infrared treatment. It is uncommon that patients will need to be reexamined in this early period after the treatment. Some physicians avoid insertion of the anoscope in the first 2 weeks after initial treatment, because injury can occur to the healing tissues.
- Pelvic sepsis can follow hemorrhoidal banding, but has not been reported after infrared treatments. Pelvic sepsis often presents with fever, rectal pain, and inability to urinate. Pelvic sepsis can result in pelvic thrombophlebitis and subsequent death. Physicians should be aware of this clinical entity, and watch for the unusual presentation in patients treated for hemorrhoidal disease.

PROCEDURE PITFALLS/COMPLICATIONS

- *Bleeding occurs during the procedure.* Rarely, IRC treatment will initiate significant bleeding from a hemorrhoid pad. Direct pressure should immediately be applied to the bleeding site with a large cotton-tipped swab. Often, the infrared coagulator tip can be activated above the bleeding site, thereby reducing blood flow into the hemorrhoid. Vigorous bleeding can also be controlled with electrocautery or the application of a rubber band to the base of the hemorrhoid.

- *The patient complains of severe pain with the procedure.* Although some investigators have touted this procedure as "painless," most patients describe a burning sensation or some discomfort. Pain is usually controlled with preprocedure ibuprofen and "verbal anesthesia." Talk to patients throughout the procedure. Warn the patient before each treatment application. Encourage a patient to "hang in there" if only one or two more applications will complete the treatment session. Some patients appreciate a brief break during the session if extensive treatment is performed. If an application is required adjacent to the dentate line, perform this treatment last. The infrared coagulator tip should never be activated distal or below the dentate line.

- *The patient requests treatment of all three hemorrhoid pads in one session.* It is uncommon for all three hemorrhoid pads to require simultaneous treatment. Patients may state that they will not return, and that treatment of all three areas should be accomplished in one setting. Treatment of the anal tissues can rarely produce an excessive scar reaction. Because anal stenosis can develop from circumferential treatment of the canal, treatment on all sides of the anal canal should be avoided.

- *The patient returns a month later and states that treatment did not work.* Patients often palpate the anal tissues after the procedure. Although external hemorrhoids may shrink after the treatment of internal hemorrhoids, external tags often persist. External tags generally do not require treatment and do not bleed. If a patient has extensive or large tags, remind him or her that they will still be present after the infrared treatment.

- *The patient returns in 18 months with redevelopment of bleeding.* The development of internal hemorrhoids is dependent on a number of lifestyle issues. Patients must be educated to increase their fresh fruit and vegetable consumption, take a daily stool bulking agent, and keep stools soft. Unfortunately, patients often revert back to their former lifestyle practices, and hemorrhoids can redevelop over time. Nevertheless, bleeding should not be assumed to be from the hemorrhoids, and colon evaluation may be needed for any patient with bleeding.

PHYSICIAN TRAINING

The IRC treatment of internal hemorrhoids is easy to learn and perform. Some skill is needed for performing anoscopy and pathology recognition in the anal canal as infrared treatments are performed through the anoscope. For physicians experienced in anoscopy, infrared treatment can be performed after just a few supervised procedures. The American Academy of Family Physicians offers workshops in the treatment of hemorrhoidal disease.

TABLE 13.1. CPT Coding for Infrared Coagulation of Internal Hemorrhoids

CPT Codes	Description	1998 Total RVUs[a]	1998 Average 50% Fees in U.S.[b]
46600	Diagnostic anoscopy, with or without collection of specimens [separate procedure]	0.81	$60
46934	Destruction of internal hemorrhoids; any method	5.44	$330

CPT only © 1998 American Medical Association. All rights reserved.

[a] Department of Health and Human Services, Health Care Financing Administration. Medicare program: revisions to payment policies and adjustments to the relative value units (RVUs) under the physician fee schedule for calendar year 1998. Federal Register 42 CFR part 414. October 31, 1997;62(211):59103–59255.

[b] 1998 Physicians' Fee Reference. West Allis, WI: Yale Wasserman, DMD, Medical Publishers, 1998.

ORDERING INFORMATION

Infrared coagulator, Ives anoscope (Redfield Corporation, 210 Summit Avenue, Montvale, NJ 07645; 800-366-1100)

K-Y jelly (Johnson and Johnson Medical, 2500 East Arbrook Boulevard, Arlington, TX 76014; 817-465-3141)

Lidocaine 5% ointment (Xylocaine ointment; Astra U.S.A., Inc., 50 Otis Street, Westborough, MA 01581; 508-366-1100)

BIBLIOGRAPHY

Ambrose NS, Morris D, Alexander-Williams J, Keighley MR. A randomized trial of photocoagulation or injection sclerotherapy for the treatment of first- and second-degree hemorrhoids. Dis Colon Rectum 1985;28:238–240.

Bat L, Melzer E, Koler M, Dreznick Z, Shemesh E. Complications of rubber band ligation of symptomatic internal hemorrhoids. Dis Colon Rectum 1993;36:287–290.

Dennison AD, Whiston RJ, Rooney S, Chadderton RD, Wherry DC, Morris DL. A randomized comparison of infrared photocoagulation with bipolar diathermy for the outpatient treatment of hemorrhoids. Dis Colon Rectum 1990;33:32–34.

Ferguson EF. Alternatives in the treatment of hemorrhoidal disease. S Med J 1988;81:606–610.

Johanson JF, Rimm A. Optimal nonsurgical treatment of hemorrhoids: a comparative analysis of infrared coagulation, rubber band ligation, and injection sclerotherapy. Am J Gastroenterol 1992;87:1600–1606.

Leicester RJ, Nicholls RJ, Chir M, Mann CV. Infrared coagulation: a new treatment for hemorrhoids. Dis Colon Rectum 1981;24:602–605.

Russel TR, Donohue JH. Hemorrhoidal banding: a warning. Dis Colon Rectum 1985;28:291–293.

Smith LE. Anal hemorrhoids [Review]. Neth J Med 1990;37(Suppl 1):S22–S32.

Templeton JL, Spence RAI, Kennedy TL, Parks TG, MacKenzie G, Hanna WA. Comparison of infrared coagulation and rubber band ligation for first and second degree haemorrhoids: a randomized prospective trial. BMJ 1983;286(6375): 1387–1389.

Zuber TJ. Anorectal disease and hemorrhoids. In: Taylor RB, ed. Manual of family practice. Boston: Little Brown, 1997:381–384.

CHAPTER 14

....

Ingrown Toenail Removal

Ingrown toenail, or onychocryptosis, is a commonly encountered problem in family practice. The condition usually presents with pain, but with progression patients experience drainage, infection, and difficulty walking. Most patients present in the second and third decades of life, but teenagers often develop ingrown toenails after they tear the corners of their toenails.

Possible causes of ingrown toenails include improperly trimmed nails, hyperhidrosis, poorly fitting footwear, trauma, subungual neoplasms, obesity, or excessive external pressure. These alterations cause the nail to improperly fit into the lateral nail groove, producing edema and inflammation of the lateral nail fold.

Stage 1 ingrown toenails are characterized by erythema, slight edema, and pain with pressure to the lateral nail fold. Stage 2 disease is marked by increased symptoms, drainage, and infection. Stage 3 ingrown toenails display magnified symptoms, granulation tissue, and lateral nail fold hypertrophy.

Many physicians advocate conservative management for stage 1 disease, such as warm soaks, cotton wick elevation of the nail corner, or antibiotics (Table 14.1). Simple partial nail avulsion has been tried for stage 2 nails, but this is only successful in eradicating the disease in 30% of patients. Stage 3 ingrown nails can develop from a laterally pointing spicule of nail beneath the nail fold. Excision of the lateral nail plate combined with lateral matricectomy is believed to provide the best chance for eradication. When treating stage 3 nails, the associated granulation tissue and lateral wall hypertrophy should also be removed.

The surgical technique of lateral nail avulsion and matricectomy has achieved the greatest success in the treatment of ingrown nails. Lateral nail excision limits the amount of nail removed, and leaves less of an area of exposed and tender nail bed. If a laterally pointing spicule of nail is found beneath the hypertrophied tissue of the lateral nail fold, remove it and create a new lateral nail edge to allow the lateral nail fold to regrow normally. The technique of wedge excision often fails to remove the spicule. Nail removal without destroying the matrix of the nail that produces lateral nail growth can permit the lateral nail to regrow beneath the lateral nail fold, producing another ingrown nail.

Historically, phenol has been used for matricectomy, but it produces

TABLE 14.1.   Management Options for Ingrown Toenails

Warm water soaks
Cotton wick insertion in the lateral groove corners
Debridement (debulking) of the lateral nail groove
Silver nitrate cautery to the hypertrophied lateral nail tissue
Complete nail avulsion
Partial nail avulsion
Wedge resection of the distal nail edge
Partial nail avulsion with
    phenol matricectomy
    sodium hydroxide matricectomy
    laser matricectomy
    electrosurgery matricectomy
Surgical excision of nail plate, nail bed, and matrix

irregular tissue destruction and can result in significant inflammation and discharge after the procedure. Laser works well for matricectomy, but is too expensive for most offices. Electrosurgery matricectomy has been demonstrated to produce consistent results, and is an easily learned technique for most family physicians.

METHODS AND MATERIALS

Patient Preparation

Patient is placed in the supine position with knees flexed (foot flat on the table) or leg extended (foot hanging off the end of the table).

Equipment

Place the following items on a drape covering the Mayo stand:

Nonsterile gloves

10-mL syringe filled with 1% lidocaine (Xylocaine), 30-gauge needle

Povidone-iodine soaked 4 × 4 gauze

1 to 2 inches of 4 × 4 gauze

Fenestrated drape

Iris scissors

Bandage scissors

2 straight hemostats

Sterile rubber band (if desired)

Nail splitter (if desired)

Monsel's solution and cotton-tipped swabs (if desired)

Electrosurgical Cart

Ellman Surgitron electrosurgical unit

2-mm and 4-mm matricectomy electrodes (flat, Teflon-coated on one side)

5-mm ball electrode

Smoke evacuator with viral particle filtering system

Items for Postprocedure Dressing

Unfolded 4 × 4 gauze (for wrapping the toe)

Antibiotic ointment

Roll of 1-inch tape

Surgical sponge slipper to wear over the bandaged toe

Telfa pad (can cut a 1-inch strip to cover the surgical site)

PROCEDURE DESCRIPTION

1. The patient is placed in the supine position, with the knees flexed (foot flat on the table) or extended (foot hanging off the end of the table). The physician wears nonsterile gloves.
2. The toe is prepped with povidone-iodine solution. A standard digital block is performed with 1% lidocaine (no epinephrine), using a 10-mL syringe and a 30-gauge needle. Usually about 2 to 3 mL on each side of the toe is sufficient for adequate anesthesia. Wait 5 to 10 minutes to allow the block to work.
3. Some physicians will use a sterile rubber band around the base of the toe for a dry operative field. A clean, unused rubber band can be placed in a sterilization pouch and put through the autoclave. Alternatively, pressure to the sides of the toes during the procedure can reduce bleeding. A tourniquet should be used only for the shortest possible time.
4. The toe is rewashed with surgical solution, and a fenestrated drape is placed over the foot, with the involved toe protruding through the drape. A nail elevator, or the closed tips of iris scissors, are slid under the cuticle to separate the nail plate from the overlying proximal nail fold.
5. The lateral one-fourth or one-fifth of the nail plate is identified as the site for the partial lateral nail removal. This is usually where the nail curves down into the toe. Use a nail splitter or bandage scissors, cutting from the distal (free) end of the nail straight back (proximally) beneath the proximal nail fold (Figs. 14.1 and 14.2). Create a straight, smooth, new lateral edge to the nail plate. When the scissors cut through the most proximal edge of the nail beneath the cuticle, a "give" can be felt.

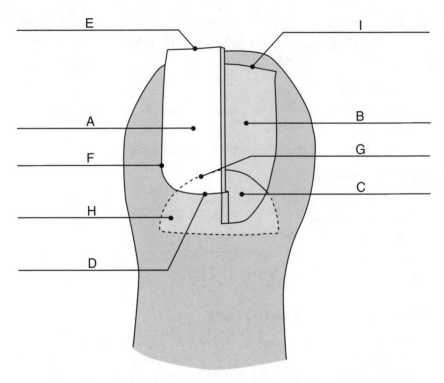

FIGURE 14.1.   Normal nail anatomy. The nail plate **(A)** receives the nutrition from the underlying nail bed **(B)**. The nail plate is created by the nail matrix **(C)**. The nail plate is visible from the proximal nail fold (cuticle) **(D)** to the distal or free edge **(E)**. The lateral nail fold lies outside of the lateral nail groove **(F)** and is where ingrown nails develop. The nail matrix can be seen at the junction with nail bed called the lunula **(G)**. Nail matrix extends out in the lateral horns **(H)**. Nail bed extends distally to the hyponychium **(I)**.

6. Grasp the lateral piece of nail with a hemostat, getting as much nail plate as possible into the teeth of the instrument. Remove the lateral nail plate, in one piece if possible, by rotating the fragment outward toward the lateral nail fold, while pulling straight out toward the end of the toe.

7. If the lateral nail plate breaks, re-grasp the remaining nail and pull it out. Make sure no fragment of nail plate remains under the proximal nail fold.

8. Electrocautery ablation is used to destroy the nail-forming matrix beneath the area where the nail plate has been removed. The flat matricectomy electrode is coated on one side to avoid damage to the overlying proximal nail fold. The electrode is placed beneath the nail fold, just above the nail bed, and cautery is applied to a bloodless field using 20 to 40 W of

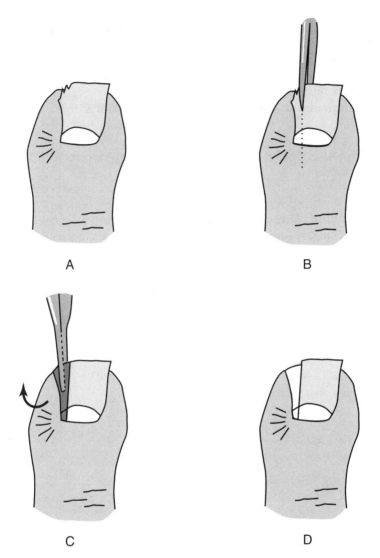

A

B

C

D

FIGURE 14.2.   Lateral nail avulsion. An ingrown nail with lateral nail fold hypertrophy is seen on the left side of the nail (**A**). After administering digital or local anesthesia, one can use scissors, a scalpel blade, or a nail splitter to cut proximally and to create a smooth, straight edge (**B**). Some physicians prefer to slide a flat nail elevator beneath the nail before making this cut in an effort to reduce nail bed trauma. The free lateral nail now is grasped with a hemostat or clamp and removed by rotating laterally while pulling out (**C**). The lateral nail bed and matrix are now exposed for ablation (**D**).

coagulation current (setting 2 to 4), with sparking produced, for two to 10 seconds, treating the entire exposed nail bed and matrix twice. A properly treated nail bed has a white appearance after electrocautery.

9. If excessive lateral granulation tissue is noted, consider removal with electrocautery ablation. A 5-mm ball electrode is moved back and forth over the lateral granulation tissue, coagulating with 40 to 50 W of current (setting 4 to 5). The destroyed tissue can usually be wiped away with gauze, and the process repeated until a concavity reveals normal tissue at the base. This site will fill in as healing takes place over the next few weeks.

10. Apply antibiotic ointment, a bulky gauze dressing, and place the patient's foot in a disposable surgical slipper. Antibiotic ointment should be applied daily until healing is complete. The patient is given the instruction sheet, and told to take ibuprofen (Motrin) and acetaminophen for postoperative pain. Daily cleansing with warm water is encouraged, and strenuous exercise is discouraged for at least one week.

TABLE 14.2. CPT Codes

CPT Codes	Description	1998 Total RVUs[a]	1998 Average 50% Fees in U.S.[b]
11730	Avulsion of nail plate, partial or complete; single	1.62	$109
11750	Excision of nail and matrix, partial or complete	4.15	$320
11752	Excision of nail and matrix, with amputation of tuft of distal phalanx	5.85	$509
11765	Wedge excision of skin of nail fold	1.25	$153

CPT only © 1998 American Medical Association. All rights reserved.
[a] Department of Health and Human Services, Health Care Financing Administration. Medicare program: revisions to payment policies and adjustments to the relative value units (RVUs) under the physician fee schedule for calendar year 1998. Federal Register 42 CFR part 414. October 31, 1997;62(211):59103–59255.
[b] 1998 Physicians' Fee Reference. West Allis, WI: Yale Wasserman, DMD, Medical Publishers, 1998.

FOLLOW UP

- A pathology evaluation performed on tissue removed during ingrown toenail surgery is rarely needed; only when an abnormal growth or suspected malignancy is encountered would a specimen be sent to the laboratory.
- If increasing pain, swelling, redness, or drainage develop, then the patient should be evaluated for infection. Infection is not uncommon after ingrown toenail removal procedures. Early intervention with oral antibiotics can be very effective in preventing infectious complications.

- Incomplete matricectomy can allow a spicule of new nail to grow laterally, interfering with the newly created lateral nail groove. A second procedure may be required to obliterate the lateral spicule if inadequate matricectomy is performed at the first procedure.

PROCEDURE PITFALLS/COMPLICATIONS

- *Prolonged application of the tourniquet can lead to distal toe ischemia.* Distal digit ischemia usually presents with duskiness, poor healing, occasional ulceration, and even necrosis. Ingrown toenail removal can be performed without a tourniquet, but it is easier with a bloodless surgical field. If a tourniquet is used, remove it as soon as possible.

- *Overaggressive electrocautery to the nail matrix can damage the underlying tissues.* Prolonged or high current cautery has the potential to damage the fascia or periosteum underlying the nail matrix. If the toe is healing poorly several weeks after the procedure, consider debridement, antibiotics, and possible x-ray evaluation.

- *The patient returns after 2 weeks with a swollen, red, inflamed toe.* Infection is not unusual after the procedure, and oral antibiotics can be liberally administered. Some practices routinely give antibiotics for a few days after the procedure. Aggressive infection management can reduce the chance of developing the rare complication of osteomyelitis.

- *The patient complains that the surgery did not get rid of the ingrown nail.* If inadequate matricectomy is performed, a spike of nail can regrow along the new lateral nail fold. This laterally growing piece of nail creates another inflammatory reaction in the lateral toe, necessitating a second procedure. The physician must make sure that the lateral horn matrix cells under the proximal nail fold are adequately ablated the first time.

- *The nail bed is lacerated when the nail is cut with the bandage scissors.* The operator must cut with the smallest blade of the scissors beneath the nail. The tips of the scissors should be slightly angled upward to avoid lacerating the fragile nail bed beneath the nail plate. Usually, bleeding from superficial lacerations is controlled by electrocautery. Deep lacerations may require suture repair and removal of additional nail.

- *The patient is surprised by the postoperative appearance of the toe.* Patients should be reminded that the procedure will permanently narrow the nail. In addition, the concavity left when the lateral granulation tissue is removed can be a shock to some individuals, but reassure the patient that the tissue will gradually fill in.

PHYSICIAN TRAINING

The technique of nail avulsion and matricectomy is easily learned by physicians with soft tissue surgery and electrosurgery experience. Physicians should have precepted patient procedures. Novice physicians may need 20 procedures before they are comfortable performing the procedure unsupervised. Experienced physicians may be comfortable after performing three to five procedures.

ORDERING INFORMATION

Ellman Surgitron electrosurgical unit, matricectomy electrodes, ball electrodes (Ellman International, 1135 Railroad Avenue, Hewlett, NY 11557; 800-835-5355)

BIBLIOGRAPHY

Benjamin RB. Excision of ingrown toenail. In: Benjamin RB, ed. Atlas of outpatient and office surgery. 2nd ed. Philadelphia: Lea & Febiger, 1994:357-359.

Ceilley RI, Collison DW. Matricectomy. J Dermatol Surg Oncol 1992;18:728-734.

Fishman HC. Practical therapy for ingrown toenails. Cutis 1983;32:159-160.

Frumkin A. Phenol cauterization of nail matrix remnants. J Dermatol Surg Oncol 1987;13:1324-1325.

Gillette RD. Practical management of ingrown toenails. Postgrad Med 1988;84:145-158.

Greenwald L, Robbins HM. The chemical matricectomy: a commentary. J Am Podiatry Assoc 1981;71:388-389.

Hettinger DF, Valinsky MS, Nuccio G, Lim R. Nail matricectomies using radio wave technique. J Am Podiatr Med Assoc 1991;81:317-321.

Leahy AL, Timon CI, Craig A, Stephens RB. Ingrowing toenails: improving treatment. Surgery 1990;107:566-567.

Quill G, Myerson M. A guide to office treatment on ingrown toenails. Hosp Med 1994;30:51-54.

Siegle RJ, Stewart R. Recalcitrant ingrowing nails. Surgical approaches [Review]. J Dermatol Surg Oncol 1992;18:744-752.

Zuber TJ, Pfenninger JL. Management of ingrown toenails. Am Fam Phys 1995;52:181-190.

CHAPTER 15

Loop Electrosurgical Excision Procedure

The loop electrosurgical excision procedure (LEEP) represents a major advance in the treatment of cervical intraepithelial neoplasia (CIN). Also known as the large loop excision of the transformation zone (LLETZ), the procedure has the advantage of providing a histologic specimen, compared with ablative procedures such as cryosurgery or laser destruction of the cervix. LEEP provides conservative management for women with cervical dysplasia, the majority of whom are in the reproductive years and desire to maintain reproductive options.

LEEP uses a fine electrosurgical wire that excises the diseased transformation zone with minimal tissue disruption and interference to the histologic analysis. The low-voltage electrical flow combines cutting and coagulation currents, thereby reducing bleeding during the procedure. Intracervical administration of local anesthetic creates good patient tolerance for this surgery. The complication rates for this office procedure are low, and patient acceptance is high.

Prendiville first reported on his experience with LEEP using large 20 × 20-mm loop electrodes. Studies have demonstrated that the greatest depth of the cervical crypts is about 7 mm deep, and that 8 mm deep electrodes are adequate to produce more than a 95% success rate in removing all diseased tissue. The original 20 mm deep electrodes removed an excessive amount of normal cervical stroma. Most LEEP procedures are performed with 15 or 20 mm-wide and 8 mm-deep electrodes.

Cervical conization can be performed with the LEEP procedure when additional removal of canal tissue is desired. After one or more passes with the electrode to remove the entire ectocervical transformation zone, an additional pass with a more narrow electrode (10 × 10 mm) can remove a cylindrical piece of upper canal tissue. Whether or not the conization is performed, most physicians performing LEEP will obtain an endocervical curettage to document that the remaining canal is free of disease.

LEEP initially was advocated for both diagnosis and treatment in one session. It soon became apparent that LEEP for all abnormal Pap smears or visually abnormal cervical appearances resulted in many women undergoing the surgical procedure unnecessarily. Patients now are selected for the procedure based upon colposcopic biopsies. Mild dysplasia is the most common neoplastic change of the cervix, and frequently undergoes spontaneous conversion back to normal. Many authors advocate LEEP only when treating ectocervical disease that has high-grade dysplasia. Low-grade dysplasia may require treatment under certain circumstances, such as patient noncompliance.

METHODS AND MATERIALS

Patient Preparation Setup

The patient should undress from the waist down, with a drape over the abdomen and legs. The patient is seated on the examination table to talk with the physician. The patient is placed in stirrups in the dorsal lithotomy position for the procedure. The adherent grounding pad is attached to the patient's thigh.

Equipment

Nonsterile Procedure Tray

Place the following items on a nonsterile drape covering the Mayo stand:

Nonsterile gloves and mask

Ring forceps

Endocervical curette

$\frac{1}{2} \times \frac{1}{2}$ inch piece of Telfa pad for removing cervical mucus after the endocervical curettage

1×1 inch piece of medium sandpaper for cleaning electrodes

Medicine cup with Lugol's (iodine) solution

Medicine cup with Monsel's paste

10 mL-syringe filled with 2% lidocaine with epinephrine (Xylocaine with epinephrine) with a needle extender and a 27-gauge, $1\frac{1}{4}$-inch needle attached

12 large cotton-tipped swabs

5 small cotton-tipped swabs

LEEP electrode: 20×8 mm

LEEP ball electrode

LEEP electrode for conization: 10×10 mm

3 pathology specimen containers with formalin

Electrosurgery Cart

Electrosurgical generator with attached electrode handpiece for the LEEP procedure, and attached grounding pad which is attached to the patient's thigh

Smoke evacuator vacuum unit attached by tubing to the coated speculum

Colposcope for Magnified Viewing/Lighting

PROCEDURE DESCRIPTION

1. The patient is placed in the dorsal lithotomy position in stirrups. The electrosurgical generator, colposcope, and smoke evacuator are plugged in and turned on. The adherent grounding pad is attached to the patient's thigh.
2. The coated speculum is inserted, and the cervix centered in the open speculum. The cervix is wiped clean with a large cotton-tipped swab. The smoke evacuator tubing is attached to the speculum.
3. Lugol's solution is applied to the cervix, staining darkly the well-glycogenated squamous tissue. The edge of the transformation zone is identified by the junction between darkly and lightly or non-staining tissue. The anesthetic is injected just outside this junction by puncturing the needle gently through the mucosa and injecting 0.5 to 2 mL in at least four sites around the cervix. Anesthetic administration should be slow, monitoring the patient for vasovagal response, or tachycardia from the anesthetic.
4. Following anesthetic administration, the cervix is wiped clean and restained with Lugol's solution. The side wall retractor is applied; avoid pinching vaginal tissue between the speculum and retractor. An appropriate sized LEEP electrode (20 mm × 8 mm) is selected, and a test pass performed to ensure adequate room for the performance of the procedure.
5. The generator is set on blend current (cut and coagulate) at 40 to 50 watts of power. The smoke evacuator is activated, and the loop electrode brought to just above the cervix at the 3 o'clock position, 2 mm lateral to the edge of staining. The electrode is activated, and inserted straight into the tissue up to the hub of the electrode. The electrode is slowly brought across the cervix, until it is 2 mm beyond the edge of staining at the 9 o'clock position. The electrode is brought straight out, and the electrode is deactivated upon leaving the cervix.
6. The ring forceps are used to grasp the tissue specimen and place it in formalin. If additional nonstaining tissue remains on the anterior and posterior lips of the cervix, then additional passes are made to remove the remaining transformation zone.
7. Once the entire transformation zone is removed, the LEEP 5 mm ball

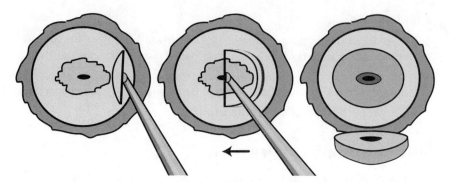

FIGURE 15.1. The loop is placed 2 to 3 mm outside of the edge of the nonstaining tissue at the 3 o'clock position, and activated just above the tissue surface. The loop is inserted straight into the tissue up to hub, and brought across the cervix at the 9 o'clock position, 2 to 3 mm beyond the edge of the nonstaining tissue at that site.

electrode is inserted into the handpiece. The generator is set at coagulation, and 50 to 60 watts of power. Cautery is applied just outside the edge of excision, and within the wound base at any bleeding sites. Good hemostasis should be achieved. Char buildup on the ball electrode can be removed with sandpaper.

8. If conization is desired, the 10 mm × 10 mm electrode is inserted into the handpiece. The generator is set on blend current at 30 to 40 watts of power. The electrode is placed into the cervical defect, 2 to 4 mm lateral to the edge of the canal, at the 3 o'clock position. The electrode is activated, and inserted up to the hub. The electrode is brought slowly across to the 9 o'clock position, just past the canal, and pulled straight out (Figs. 15.1 and 15.2). The electrode is deactivated as it leaves the cervical tissue. The endocervical specimen is grasped with the ring forceps, and placed in its own formalin container. Any additional bleeding sites are controlled with the ball cautery.

9. An endocervical curettage is performed to exclude disease in the remaining canal. Once the curette has passed within the canal, the mucus from the canal is removed with the ring forceps and squeezed onto a small piece of Telfa. The Telfa is placed in the formalin container with the specimen from the curette. The pathologist can centrifuge the cells free from the Telfa.

10. Monsel's paste is placed within the wound base, using a large cotton-tipped applicator. Good hemostasis again is confirmed. The smoke evacuator tubing is removed from the speculum, and the speculum slowly removed from the vagina. Any solutions that have drained onto the vulva are wiped clear. The grounding pad is removed from the patient's thigh.

FOLLOW UP

- Patients are asked to return for a Pap smear in 4 months. Examination of the cervix before 3 months have elapsed often reveals reactive or reparative changes. Reparative changes may appear acetowhite under the colposcope or cause false-positive readings on the Pap smear. While some anxious patients may request an earlier examination for peace of mind, early examinations are discouraged.
- Following the Pap smear at 4 months, the patient is re-examined under the colposcope in 8 months to determine if there is the presence of residual disease. Some authors believe there should be a disease-free interval (1 year) before dysplasia is recognized again, for recurrent disease to be present.
- Atypia or mild dysplasia often is detected in the first year following LEEP. These minor changes appear much more often in women who continue smoking. Women with human papillomavirus (HPV), or those who require LEEP, must be effectively counseled about the deleterious effects of cigarette smoking on the immune system environment of the cervix.
- There are conflicting recommendations in medical literature regarding the management of positive margins in the LEEP specimens. The management may take into consideration several issues, including the degree of dysplasia and which margin is involved. Lateral margins that are positive may not require immediate re-excision, as the ball cautery eliminates an additional 5 mm of lateral tissue. Deep margins may require immediate re-excision, especially if high-grade dysplasia is involved. Many authors have performed

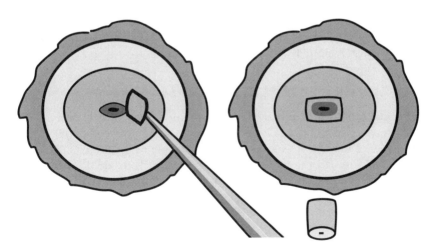

FIGURE 15.2. The conization is performed, when needed, by placing the 10 × 10 mm loop in the LEEP base adjacent to the canal at the 3 o'clock position. The loop is inserted to the hub, and brought across the canal, exiting at the 9 o'clock position.

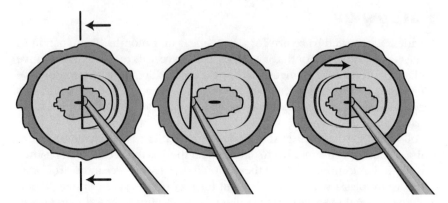

FIGURE 15.3. If the loop stalls halfway across the cervix, the loop should be deactivated. The loop is withdrawn at the 3 o'clock position. The loop is placed 2 to 3 mm outside of the non-staining tissue at the 9 o'clock position, activated and inserted to the hub, and brought across the cervix to join up with the prior excision path that had started at the 3 o'clock position.

immediate repeat LEEP, only to retrieve normal tissue. There may be many reasons why the re-excision fails to obtain dysplastic tissue. The inflammatory response to the original procedure may effectively eliminate any residual diseased tissue.

- Consider immediate repeat LEEP when high-grade dysplasia is present in the deep surgical margin. If the physician and patient choose to follow up for persisting disease, frequent examinations and Pap smears (every 3 to 4 months) are advised. Pap smears have a high (20–30%) false-negative rate, and should be repeated often to offset this error. Low-grade changes at a lateral margin may be followed with frequent cytology.

PROCEDURE PITFALLS/COMPLICATIONS

- ***The electrode gets stuck when passing through the cervix.*** The electrode can get bogged down as it passes through the cervix (Fig. 15.3.). The power may be set too low for the procedure, or the electrode may be pulled through the tissue too quickly. If the electrode does get stuck, it should be deactivated and brought out along the same path it traveled (pull it out at 3:00). The electrode is placed above the tissue on the opposite side (at 9:00), activated, and slowly brought across the cervix to meet the first electrode path.

- ***Blood sprayed out of the vagina during the procedure.*** Rare reports of this type of bleeding have been noted. While this is uncommon, it is suggested that physicians wear a mask to cover the mucous membranes. Physicians should also consider eye protection for this procedure.

- *The patient passed out during the procedure.* Vasovagal reactions are common when procedures are performed on the cervix. Most vasovagal reactions occur following administration of the anesthetic. If patients become lightheaded, diaphoretic, or nauseated, then consider elevating the legs (lifting them out of the stirrups) to improve cerebral blood flow.

- *The patient experienced a burn on the inner thigh before the procedure.* There are a number of machines, tubes, and wires associated with this procedure. Novice physicians are often looking at the machines instead of the patient. In preparation for the procedure, the physician may activate the electrode while holding it near the upper inner thigh, while simultaneously looking at the machines. Physicians are urged to only activate the electrode when looking directly at the tip.

- *The pathologist reports excessive tissue artifact in the specimens.* If the electrosurgical generator is set too high, excessive burn artifact can occur. The generator should be set at 40 to 50 watts of power for ectocervical excisions. The generator power can be decreased if excessive tissue burning is noted. The power is reduced for endocervical excisions (conization).

- *Excessive bleeding is noted following the procedure.* Application of Monsel's paste to the wound bed can reduce postoperative bleeding. Late bleeding usually develops 2 to 10 days following the procedure. Late bleeding has been noted to occur following intercourse, straining, or vigorous physical exercise.

PHYSICIAN TRAINING

Colposcopy skills are considered a prerequisite to the performance of the LEEP procedure. Most physicians perform LEEP with the aid of the colposcope. Proper surgical skills also may be a prerequisite; rarely suture ligature may be needed. Physicians skilled in skin electrosurgery find LEEP a fairly easy technique to learn. It is recommended that those skilled in electrosurgery

TABLE 15.1. CPT Codes for LEEP Procedure

CPT Codes	Description	1998 Total RVUs[a]	1998 Average 50% Fees in U.S.[b]
57460	Colposcopy with LEEP	5.31	$748
57522	Conization by LEEP	7.54	$725

CPT only © 1998 American Medical Association. All rights reserved.

[a] Department of Health and Human Services, Health Care Financing Administration. Medicare program: revisions to payment policies and adjustments to the relative value units (RVUs) under the physician fee schedule for calendar year 1998. Federal Register 42 CFR part 414. October 31, 1997;62(211):59103–59255.

[b] 1998 Physicians' Fee Reference. West Allis, WI: Yale Wasserman, DMD, Medical Publishers, 1998.

perform at least 10 supervised procedures before attempting the procedure unsupervised. Family physicians should seek out peers who are experienced in LEEP to serve as preceptors.

ORDERING INFORMATION

Kevorkian curette without basket, Vu-More coated large speculums and coated side-wall retractors, Lugol's iodine solution, AstrinGyn (Monsel's paste), LEEP 6000 generator, smoke evacuator system, connector tubing, LEEP electrodes, adherent grounding pads (Cooper Surgical, 15 Forest Parkway, Shelton, CT 06484; 800-848-0033)

Needle extender 5 inch (Premier Medical Products, 3600 Horizon Drive, King of Prussia, PA 19406; 888-773-6872)

BIBLIOGRAPHY

Bigrigg A, Haffenden DK, Sheehan AL, Codling BW, Read MD. Efficacy and safety of large-loop excision of the transformation zone. Lancet 1994;343:32–34.

Chappatte OA, Byrne DL, Raju KS, Nayagum M, Kenney A. Histologic differences between colposcopic-directed biopsy and loop excision of the transformation zone (LETZ): a cause for concern. Gynecol Oncol 1991;43:46–50.

Ferris DG, Hainer BL, Pfenninger JL, Zuber TJ, DeWitt DE, Line RL. Electrosurgical loop excision of the cervical transformation zone: the experience of family physicians. J Fam Pract 1995;41:337–344.

Howe DT, Vincenti AC. Is large loop excision of the transformation zone (LLETZ) more accurate than colposcopically directed punch biopsy in the diagnosis of cervical intraepithelial neoplasia? Br J Obstet Gynecol 1991;98:588–591.

Kainz C, Tempfer C, Sliutz G, Breitenecker G, Reinthaller A. Radiosurgery in the management of cervical intraepithelial neoplasia. J Reprod Med 1996;41:409–414.

Prendiville W, Cullimore J, Norman S. Large loop excision of the transformation zone (LLETZ). A new method of management for women with cervical intraepithelial neoplasia. Br J Obstet Gynecol 1989;96:1054–1060.

Randall T. Loop electrosurgical excision procedures gaining acceptance for cervical intraepithelial neoplasia. JAMA 1991;266:460–462.

Whiteley PF, Olah KS. Treatment of cervical intraepithelial neoplasia: experience with the low-voltage diathermy loop. Am J Obstet Gynecol 1990;162:1272–1277.

Wright TC, Gagnon S, Ferenczy A, Richart RM. Excising CIN lesions by loop electrosurgical procedure. Contemp Obstet Gynecol 1991;36:57–74.

Wright TC, Gagnon S, Richart RM, Ferenczy A. Treatment of cervical intraepithelial neoplasia using the loop electrosurgical excision procedure. Obstet Gynecol 1992;79:173–178.

CHAPTER 16
....

No-Scalpel Vasectomy

Vasectomy is a simple, relatively inexpensive, and effective form of permanent contraception. About 500,000 vasectomy procedures are performed annually in the United States. The procedure is well-suited to the office setting, and takes about 15 to 30 minutes to perform.

The no-scalpel vasectomy technique represents a major improvement in surgical sterilization. The technique is less invasive, less time consuming, and produces fewer complications. Because there is no incision, no-scalpel vasectomy is believed to decrease men's fears about the procedure. Infection and bleeding rates also appear to be lower with this procedure.

The no-scalpel vasectomy technique uses a small (2- to 3-mm) midline puncture into the scrotum using a special sharp-tipped instrument (vas dissection forceps). The three-finger isolation technique (left thumb and index finger on top, left middle finger beneath the scrotum) swings the vas deferens to below the puncture site, allowing the forceps, held in the right hand, to elevate the vas through the tiny puncture. Once the vas deferens has been isolated from all other tissues, a short (¼- to ½-inch) segment of the tube is removed. The cut ends of the vas are sealed using a battery cautery, which produces fewer sperm granulomas and less chance of recanalization than electrosurgical (hyfrecator) or suture ligation techniques of vas end closure. The cut ends of the vas are separated by using a small metal clip on the fascial tissues, thereby reducing the chances of spontaneous recanalization and procedure failure.

One argument for removing a small portion of vas deferens at the time of the surgery is the visual confirmation provided to the patient. Vas segments do not need to be sent to the pathologist after completing the procedure. The histologic confirmation of the vas is expensive, and does not confirm the procedure's success. The segments are placed in formalin and should be kept by the patient until two postoperative semen examinations are obtained. In the rare event that the semen examinations do not clear, the segments of tube can be histologically examined to ensure that the surgeon actually removed vas deferens. Semen examinations are very important, and are provided free to patients. Two specimen containers for semen samples are given to the patient at the time of the operation.

Good local anesthetic technique produces pain-free procedures for most patients. Following local anesthesia in the midline scrotal skin, external spermatic sheath injection is performed for vasal nerve block. The method introduces the local anesthetic around the vas and vasal nerves, after three-finger isolation of the vas deferens, producing good anesthesia at a site above the surgical site. This technique provides superior results and is more popular with patients than older anesthetic techniques.

Proper preprocedure counseling is critical to a satisfactory procedure outcome. Patients should never be pressured into a decision for permanent sterilization. Studies suggest that up to 10% of couples may express regret after permanent sterilization. Proper counseling may deter individuals in an unstable relationship from undergoing a procedure they will regret at a later date, and can also reduce the physician's legal liability. All patients and spouses (or significant others) are scheduled for a 30-minute preprocedure counseling session and viewing of a patient education videotape.

METHODS AND MATERIALS

Patient Preparation

The procedure trays are prepared before the patient is brought to the procedure room. Some practices have the nurse wait outside the room during the procedure to reduce patient discomfort. The patient should get undressed from the waist down and place a sheet over the legs. An absorbent sheet is placed beneath the patient. The patient is then placed in the supine position for the procedure, with the legs extended and slightly separated.

Equipment

Nonsterile Tray for Anesthesia/Postoperative Care

Place the following items on a nonsterile sheet covering the Mayo stand:

Nonsterile gloves

Povidone-iodine solution soaked into 4×4 gauze (in a sterile basin)

10-mL syringe filled with 1% lidocaine (Xylocaine), and a 25-gauge 1¼-inch needle

Antibiotic ointment

2 inches of nonsterile 4×4 gauze

Patient-supplied athletic supporter

2 postoperative semen collection containers (in a plastic bag)

Formalin container for the excised portions of vas deferens

Basin with sterile saline poured onto 1 inch of 4×4 gauze

Sterile Procedure Tray

Place the following items on a sterile sheet covering the Mayo stand:

Sterile gloves

Sterile fenestrated drape

Sterile nonfenestrated drape

Vas dissecting forceps

Atraumatic vas clamp

Disposable battery cautery unit placed inside of a sterile glove

2 inches of sterile 4 × 4 gauze

2 pair of straight hemostats

1 curved hemostat

Surgical clip (Hemoclip) applicator

1 container (clip) of medium metal surgical clips (Hemoclips)

Iris scissors

PROCEDURE DESCRIPTION

1. The patient is placed in the supine position on the table, with the legs extended and slightly separated. The scrotum, penis, and inner upper thigh areas are liberally washed with povidone-iodine solution. The physician approaches the scrotum from the patient's right side. The three-finger technique (Fig. 16.1) is used to swing the right vas deferens immediately below the median raphe on the upper portion of the anterior scrotum.

2. About 1 to 2 mL of 1% lidocaine is injected into the skin over the median raphe. The needle then is inserted cephalad until the tip is parallel and adjacent to the right vas deferens, near the upper portion of the scrotum. About 2 to 4 mL of anesthetic is injected. The external spermatic sheath block is accomplished. The needle is withdrawn. The physician turns to face the patient's feet. The three-finger technique is applied (upside down) to the left scrotum, swinging the left vas beneath the anesthetized midline skin. The needle is inserted along the left vas deferens, and the left side is anesthetized similarly. The needle is withdrawn.

3. Some physicians reapply povidone-iodine solution to the scrotum. The physician wears sterile gloves. The penis is lifted upward and laid on the lower abdominal wall. The fenestrated drape is placed, with the scrotum protruding through the fenestration, and the penis held in the upward position by the overlying drape. A nonfenestrated drape is placed distal to the first drape, and between the patient's legs.

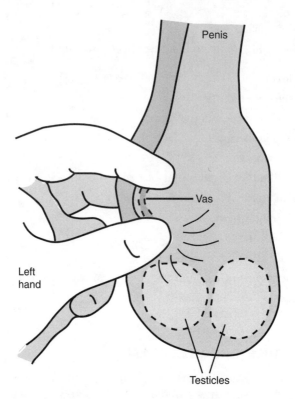

FIGURE 16.1. The three-finger technique. The left thumb and index finger are on top of the scrotum and the left middle finger is below. The vas is isolated and swung beneath the median raphe of the scrotum.

4. The three-finger technique isolates the right vas deferens beneath the anesthetized midline skin. The vas clamp is applied, holding the right vas just beneath the scrotal skin. The vas clamp is rotated upward, with the handle placed on the lower abdominal wall. A 2-mm puncture is made into the skin, just above the vas and distal to the vas clamp, using the sharp-tipped vas dissecting forceps. The tips of the vas dissecting forceps stretch the skin, and then spread the tissues down to the vas wall. The tips of the instrument are opened, with the curve directed down to the scrotum, and the right tip puncturing the wall of the vas. The tips are then rotated upward by turning the right palm upward, and the vas dissecting forceps elevate the vas up through the skin puncture.

5. The vas dissecting forceps continue to hold the vas above the scrotum. The left hand releases the vas clamp from the scrotum, and the clamp immediately grasps the elevated loop of the vas. The tips of the atraumatic

vas clamp should be directly onto the center of the wall of the vas. These maneuvers must be performed carefully to avoid dropping the vas back into the scrotum. A loop of vas is held elevated above the scrotal skin.

6. The vas dissecting forceps are used to separate the vas from the surrounding fascia, vessels, and tissue. The fascia is pushed downward by spreading the tips of the forceps open, leaving only the vas in the clamp.

7. Two cuts are made with the Iris scissors halfway across the vas (hemi-transection). The cut is made low (near the fascia) on the proximal (testicular) loop of the vas, and the cut is made high (near the clamp) on the distal (abdominal) loop of the vas (Fig. 16.2). The tip of the battery cautery unit is placed within the vas lumen below each hemi-transection (in the portions of vas extending into the scrotum that will remain inside the body after the procedure). The cautery is activated for 1 to 3 seconds until tissue coagulation occurs and the center of each tube has turned white. A full thickness burn through the entire wall of the vas is not desirable. The battery cautery unit is withdrawn.

8. The fascia near the proximal (testicular) cut is grasped and elevated with one or two hemostats. The Iris scissors complete the cut through the proximal vas, and the transected testicular end slips down into the scrotum between the clamps holding the fascia. The other end of the vas is still held by the vas clamp. A metal medium Hemoclip is applied over the fascia and up to the distal end of the vas (Fig. 16.3). The vas itself is not clamped by the Hemoclip. Try to include the vas artery (immediately adjacent to the vas) in the clamp, thereby creating good hemostasis while also interposing fascia between the cut ends of the vas.

9. Once the Hemoclip has been applied, the second transection of the vas is completed. The ¼- to ½-inch piece of vas still held by the vas clamp is placed in formalin. The distal cut end of the vas should protrude above the fascial clip. The vas is inspected one more time to ensure good hemostasis. All instruments are removed, and the right vas is returned to the scrotum.

10. The physician pivots, now facing the patient's feet. The three-finger technique is used to isolate the left vas deferens beneath the center of the scrotal skin. The vas clamp is placed inside the small skin puncture, and it grasps the left vas. The left vas is elevated through the small skin puncture site. The left vas now is held as a loop above the scrotal skin.

11. The left vas is treated in the same fashion as the right side. Once the left side is completed, the skin is checked for hemostasis. Saline on gauze is used to wash off the povidone-iodine solution from the patient. Antibiotic ointment is placed on the wound, and dry gauze applied over the site. The athletic supporter is placed while the patient is still lying supine, being sure to comfortably position the gauze inside the sup-

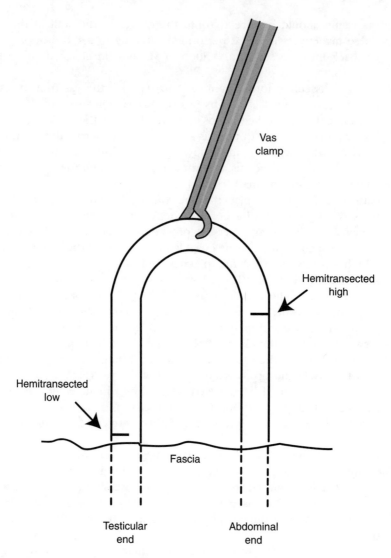

Vas
clamp

Hemitransected
high

Hemitransected
low

Fascia

Testicular
end

Abdominal
end

FIGURE 16.2. The atraumatic vas clamp grasps the middle of the loop of the vas above the scrotal skin. The sites of hemitransection for the testicular and abdominal ends are shown.

porter. The patient is slowly raised to a seated position, and briefly observed for dizziness, before being permitted to dress. The patient is given the two empty semen specimen containers, and the sections of vas in formalin (to be held until the postoperative semen specimens are clear).

FOLLOW UP

- If a patient's first semen check contains just a few sperm, the examination should be repeated in 2 to 4 weeks. Sometimes residual sperm exist in the distal vas (beyond the site of the vasectomy), and additional ejaculations are needed to clear the remaining sperm.
- If the second semen check still demonstrates large numbers of motile sperm, the surgeon probably failed to correctly identify one or both vas deferens at the time of the vasectomy. Inexperienced physicians can be confused by other scrotal structures (muscle). Physicians often wonder about an accessory vas as the cause for persisting sperm in the ejaculate. However, a third vas is a very rare finding, and most primary failures relate to surgical technique. A second attempt at the surgery can be performed, although a more experienced physician may be consulted before the second attempt.
- Late failures do occur. It is hoped that if recanalization occurs, it will develop early enough to be identified by the postoperative semen examinations. We delay the first semen check for 20 ejaculations in an attempt to clear the vas. The second specimen is checked 6 weeks later (after about 40 ejaculations). Rare occurrences of late failure have been documented, but most physicians do not perform annual semen checks to discover the rare late failure.
- Sperm granulomas are dilations or blow-outs of the cut ends of the vas. Sperm granulomas can become fairly large, and may be tender if the nearby

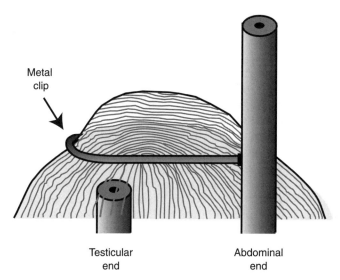

FIGURE 16.3. The metal clip secures the fascia over the testicular end. The clip goes up but not across the abdominal end of the vas.

TABLE 16.1.   CPT Codes

CPT Codes	Description	1998 Total RVUs[a]	1998 Average 50% Fee in U.S[b]
55250	Vasectomy [separate procedure]	6.20	$500

[a] Department of Health and Human Services, Health Care Financing Administration. Medicare program: revisions to payment policies and adjustments to the relative value units (RVUs) under the physician fee schedule for calendar year 1998. Federal Register 42 CFR part 414. October 31, 1997;62(211):59103–59255.
[b] 1998 Physicians' Fee Reference. West Allis, WI: Yale Wasserman, DMD, Medical Publishers, 1998.

vas nerves are incorporated into the expanding wall of the granuloma. Sperm granulomas generally do not require needle drainage, as they resolve over time. Anti-inflammatory medications may be beneficial in reducing swelling and discomfort associated with sperm granulomas.

PROCEDURE PITFALLS/COMPLICATIONS

• *The patient experiences chronic aching just above the testicle for months after the procedure.* Chronic testicular discomfort either after sexual intercourse or unrelated to intercourse is a recognized complication of vasectomy. Obstruction of the vas deferens results in a buildup of pressure, causing epididymal engorgement and, occasionally, epididymal blow-outs. Epididymal enlargement is noted by ultrasound in nearly 50% of patients, resolving in nearly all patients over several months. Men should be advised of this usually self-limiting problem, especially those under the age of 30 years of age who can generate significant intraluminal pressure during ejaculation.

• *The patient develops bruising of the scrotal skin and marked swelling of the scrotum after the procedure.* Hematoma formation usually results from bleeding in the scrotal wall, or from bleeding from the vasal artery. Some bruising of the scrotal skin may occur with the procedure, and should not create excessive concern. Hematoma formation within the scrotum should be avoided because large scrotal hematomas may require surgical drainage. Most hematomas resolve spontaneously. Once the vas has been cut, the local fascia can be lifted over the proximal end of the vas, and a Hemoclip placed over the fascia. This clip is applied up to the distal vas, and can clamp the vasal artery and vein, which are adjacent to the vas. A properly placed clip can create a bloodless field. The surgical site should always be closely examined for adequate hemostasis before the vas is returned to the scrotum.

• *The patient complains of pain in the right side throughout the procedure.* Good anesthetic technique usually results in a pain-free procedure. Some physicians report greater difficulty in anesthetizing the right side. The reasons for this are not entirely clear, but additional anesthetic or a second administration to the right side (just before starting the procedure) can be performed.

* *The patient's ejaculate has sperm present years after previously being clear.* Late failures are very rare, but can occur. It is believed that recanalization develops between the cut ends of the vas, and that sperm travel through the new channel. It is hoped that by transposing the fascia between the cut ends of the vas, that recanalization is much less likely to occur.

* *A tender nodule develops in the scrotum after the procedure.* A sperm granuloma can develop at the cut end of the vas, or in the epididymis. Sperm granulomas are believed to be "blow-outs" that develop from increased intraluminal pressure in the muscular vas. Sperm granulomas are more common after suture ligation or electrosurgical cauterization of the cut vas. Battery (thermal) cautery is used because it appears to produce fewer sperm granulomas. Sperm granulomas generally do not need to be drained with a needle as they resolve spontaneously with time.

PHYSICIAN TRAINING

Physicians should receive formal education in the no-scalpel vasectomy technique, both as part of a formal course or workshop, and with supervised patient experience. The illustrated guide or videotapes available from the Association for Voluntary Surgical Contraception (AVSC) provide excellent step-by-step instruction; however, most training physicians were only able to master about 80% of the no-scalpel techniques without hands-on instruction. Even long-time vasectomists had difficulty with the newer techniques. Many physicians skilled in no-scalpel vasectomy are available to provide precepted experience. AVSC provides a list of potential preceptors. It is uncommon that a physician can confidently provide vasectomy services without at least 10 precepted procedures.

ORGANIZATIONS PROVIDING EDUCATION, INFORMATION, VIDEOTAPES, AND INSTRUMENTS FOR NO-SCALPEL VASECTOMY

Advanced Meditech International, 86-38 53rd Avenue, Suite 100, Flushing, NY 11373; 800-635-2452

Association for Voluntary Surgical Contraception (AVSC), 79 Madison Avenue, New York, NY 10016; 212-561-8000

Patient Education Videotape: Plainly Creative Works, 809 Elm Street, Essexville, MI 48732; 800-462-2492

ORDERING INFORMATION

Hemoclip applicator and medium Hemoclips (Weck Corporation, 11311 Concept Boulevard, Largo, FL 33773; 800-237-0169)

Vas clamp, vas dissecting forceps, and battery cautery (Advanced Meditech International, 86-38 53rd Avenue, Suite 100, Flushing, NY 11373; 800-635-2452)

BIBLIOGRAPHY

Alderman PM. Complications in a series of 1224 vasectomies. J Fam Pract 1991;33:579-584.

Esho J, Cass AS. Recanalization rate following method of vasectomy using interposition of fascial sheath of vas deferens. J Urol 1978;120:178-179.

Goldstein M. No-scalpel vasectomy: a kinder, gentler approach. Patient Care 1994;28:55-73.

Gonzales B, Marston-Ainley S, Vansintejan G, Li PS. No-scalpel vasectomy: an illustrated guide for surgeons. New York: Association for Voluntary Surgical Contraception, 1992.

Li PS, Li SQ, Schlegel PN, Goldstein M. External spermatic sheath injection for vasal nerve block. Urology 1992;39:173-176.

Li SQ, Goldstein M, Zhu J, Huber D. No-scalpel vasectomy. J Urol 1991;145:341-344.

Miller WB, Shain RN, Pasta DJ. The pre- and post-sterilization regret in husbands and wives. J Nerv Ment Dis 1991;179:602-608.

Rajfer J, Bennett CJ. Vasectomy. Urol Clin North Am 1988;15:631-634.

Schmidt SS, Minckler TM. The vas after vasectomy: comparison of cauterization methods. Urology 1992;40:468-470.

Stockton MD, Davis LE, Bolton KM. No-scalpel vasectomy: a technique for family physicians. Am Fam Physician 1992;46:1153-1164.

Zuber TJ. Association between vasectomy and prostate cancer. Consultant 1994;34:151-152.

CHAPTER 17

. . . .

Skin Cryosurgery

Cryosurgery causes controlled destruction of benign, premalignant, and malignant skin growths. During freezing, heat is rapidly withdrawn from the target tissue or lesion using a probe tip that contains a refrigerant liquid. Human tissue freezes at $-2.2°C$, and actual tissue destruction usually begins between $-10°C$ and $-20°C$. Most closed-probe systems using nitrous oxide can achieve temperatures in the probe tip between $-65°C$ and $-89°C$.

An iceball is created in the tissue during cryosurgery. The edge of the iceball achieves a temperature of $0°C$, which is not cold enough for tissue destruction. The tissue at this edge usually recovers. The edge of the iceball should extend 2 to 3 mm beyond the edge of the lesion being destroyed. Most investigators advocate a freeze-thaw-freeze technique, as greater cell death is achieved in tissue previously frozen. Because iceball formation is geometric in all directions, the lateral extent of the iceball gives a good estimation of the depth of the destruction.

Cryosurgery is anesthetic to the tissue being treated. Most patients do not require anesthesia for this procedure. Many patients experience a burning sensation during or after cryosurgery, but generally the discomfort of an injected anesthetic exceeds the discomfort of skin cryosurgery.

Some of the many lesions amenable to cryotherapy are listed in Tables 17.1 and 17.2. Cryosurgery has been most extensively used for the treatment of actinic keratoses. Cryosurgery provides rapid destruction of multiple keratoses, and is more cost-effective than surgical therapy of many individual lesions. Many insurers now require an initial treatment with chemotherapy (5-fluorouracil) before reimbursing for cryosurgery of actinic keratoses.

Primary skin cancers have been demonstrated to have cure rates in excess of 95% after cryosurgery. Ultrasound scans have been used as a guide to cancer depth and cryosurgery treatment time, but some centers advocate the use of temperature probes or shave excision and curettage before cryosurgery of skin cancer. Most of the medical literature suggests that cryosurgery be limited to the treatment of non-melanoma skin cancers; however, the technique has been demonstrated to be effective therapy for the premalignant lesion lentigo maligna.

Cryosurgery is a safe, effective, and time-efficient office treatment for a wide variety of skin lesions. The relative contraindications (Table 17.3) and

149

TABLE 17.1. Lesions for Which Cryosurgery Is the Treatment of Choice

Actinic keratoses
Dermatofibroma
Leukoplakia
Mucocele of the lip
Pyogenic granuloma
Sebaceous hyperplasia
Superficial basal cell carcinoma
Verrucae

Adapted from Torre D. Cutaneous cryosurgery: current state of the art. J Dermatol Surg Oncol 1985;11:292.

TABLE 17.2. Lesions for Which Cryosurgery Is an Alternative Treatment or a Recommended Combination Therapy

Abscess
Acne pits and scars
Acne cysts
Acrochordon
Angiomas
Angiofibromas
Basal cell carcinoma
Bowen's disease
Chloasma
Condyloma acuminata
Cylindroma
Eosinophilic granuloma
Erythroplasia of Queyrat
Granuloma annulare
Hidadrenoma
Hidadrenitis
Hypertrophic scars
Hyperpigmentation
Keloid
Lentigo maligna
Molluscum contagiosum
Neurofibroma
Rhinophyma
Sarcoidosis of the skin
Seborrheic keratoses
Squamous cell carcinoma
Syringoma
Trichoepithelioma
Verrucae plana (flat warts)
Verrucae plantaris
Wrinkles of the skin

Adapted from Torre D. Cutaneous cryosurgery: current state of the art. J Dermatol Surg Oncol 1985;11:292.

TABLE 17.3. Relative Contraindications to Cryosurgery

Active syphilis infection
Active, severe collagen vascular disease
Active, severe cytomegalovirus infection
Active, severe Epstein-Barr virus infection
Active, severe subacute bacterial endocarditis
Active, severe ulcerative colitis
Acute poststreptococcal glomerulonephritis
Chronic, severe hepatitis B infection
High serum levels of cryoglobulin
High-dose steroid medication treatment
Immunoproliferative neoplasms, myelomas, lymphomas
Macroglobulinemia

Adapted from Hocutt JE. Skin cryosurgery for the family physician. Am Fam Physician 1993;48:445–452.

complications are few, and this technique has been a trusted friend of the family physician for many years. Although some physicians prefer liquid nitrogen applied with a cotton swab, the use of closed-probe nitrous oxide systems can provide more controlled destruction, and may be more cost-effective because of the evaporative loss with liquid nitrogen.

METHODS AND MATERIALS

Patient Preparation

The patient is seated or lying down comfortably. The area to be treated is exposed and cleaned, if needed.

Equipment

Place the following items on a nonsterile drape covering the Mayo stand:

Nonsterile gloves
1 inch of 4×4 gauze
1 inch of water-soluble jelly (K-Y)
Dermal tips for the cryosurgery unit
Antibiotic ointment
Bandage
Cryosurgical Treatment Unit
Cryosurgical tank with the attached administration unit ("cryogun")

PROCEDURE DESCRIPTION

1. The areas to be treated are examined, and the skin cleared of debris or dirt. Anesthesia can be performed for selected deep or tender (e.g., periungual) areas, but generally is not required as the freezing produces an anesthetic effect. Hyperkeratotic lesions can be shaved down with a No. 15 blade to enhance the ability of cryosurgery to achieve adequate tissue destruction.
2. A proper sized cryosurgical tip should be selected. The tip should approximate the size of the target lesion as closely as possible. The tip should be firmly attached to the cryogun to prevent leakage of nitrous oxide.
3. A water-soluble gel is applied to the tip for thermal conductivity. The tip is positioned vertically onto the target skin lesion with the cryotip *at ambient temperature*. The cryogun is activated, causing the gel to turn white. The duration of the freeze depends on the time required to cause the iceball (the white appearance of the tissue) to extend 2 to 3 mm out from the edge of the lesion (Fig. 17.1).
4. Once an adequate freeze has been obtained, the cryogun is deactivated. As the instrument tip and the lesion thaw, the white color of the gel clears. The cryotip now is removed from the patient.
5. The treatment site is thawed, and the tissue turns from white iceball to red in color (Fig. 17.2). Thawing of vascular lesions, such as pyogenic granulomas, can produce vigorous bleeding. Direct pressure can be applied for hemostasis. A repeat freeze is performed after the thawing of the tissue.

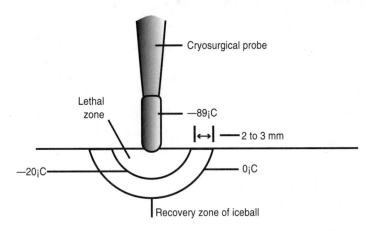

FIGURE 17.1. Cryosurgical probe placed on the skin. The iceball extends deep into the tissue roughly the same distance that it extends laterally from the probe. The edge of the iceball cools only to 0°C. Therefore the iceball should extend 2 to 3 mm beyond the lesion to be destroyed.

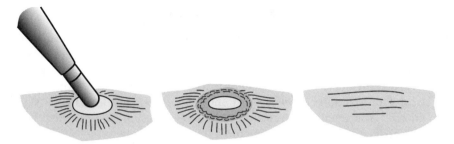

FIGURE 17.2.   Following treatment, the iceball thaws, and erythema and swelling are noted. The area often heals with very good cosmetic results.

6. Once the procedure is completed, antibiotic ointment and a bandage are applied to the treatment site.

FOLLOW UP

- When properly performed, cryosurgery is relatively free of serious complications. Most patients do not require routine wound follow up. Some patients are concerned about hemorrhagic blisters immediately after cryosurgery, or erythematous skin changes at the treatment site in the first month after the procedure. Blisters can be drained for symptom relief, and patients can be reassured that the treatment area generally turns white with time.
- Patients with human papillomavirus (HPV)-related verrucous lesions can be rechecked in 6 to 8 weeks for treatment success. If the lesion persists or regrows, re-treatment can be accomplished at that time. Warts that are frozen can transform into "ring warts" (a rim of warty tissue that encircles the site of a previously treated wart). Adequate freezing times can reduce, but not completely eliminate, the risk that ring warts will develop.
- Cancerous or precancerous lesions usually are reexamined in 1 and 6 months after therapy to document treatment success. Nodular tissue that is present at the treatment site of a previous skin cancer could represent scar formation or cancer regrowth. Nodular tissue in this setting can be considered for biopsy or re-treatment.
- Some patients, such as those with circulating cryoglobulins, have an exaggerated response to cryosurgery (excessive scar reaction, excessive blistering, or skin necrosis in excess of that expected). These patients often exhibit other immune-related disorders, such as those listed in Table 17.3. If the wound develops excessive blistering, pain, skin breakdown, or sloughing, it should receive extensive postoperative care to ensure the best possible outcome.

PROCEDURE PITFALLS/COMPLICATIONS

• *The patient developed persisting numbness in the finger after cryosurgery.* Cryosurgery can damage subcutaneous nerves, especially when performed on the digits. Although the nerve sheath is relatively resistant to freezing, the nerve axon is susceptible to damage. During the cryosurgical treatment, traction can be applied once the tip has developed good skin contact. The traction elevates the skin and the lesion being treated, and may reduce damage to the structures beneath the skin.

• *The patient developed hypopigmentation at the treatment site.* Cryosurgery can be toxic to melanocytes, and can result in permanent hypopigmentation. Cryosurgery is often used in the treatment of skin hyperpigmentation. Lesions that are on cosmetically important areas of the body, such as the face, should be treated cautiously. African-Americans and other dark-skinned individuals can be considered for alternate therapies.

• *An area of full thickness skin necrosis developed after cryotherapy.* Certain conditions can predispose the patient to an exaggerated response to the freezing of the skin. Patients with conditions that can produce serum cold-induced antibodies (cryoglobulins) are at greatest risk for marked skin necrosis after cryosurgery. Some of these conditions are listed in Table 17.3 and include neoplasms, collagen vascular diseases, severe viral illnesses, and inflammatory conditions. Patients with these conditions can be pretreated in the axilla to predict the response to cryosurgery.

• *The vascular lesion pyogenic granuloma persisted after cryosurgery.* Certain vascular, pigmented, and fibrous lesions can be resistant to cryosurgery. Vascular lesions contain warm blood, which resists heat transfer and cryosurgical destruction. Although pyogenic granulomas do respond well to cryosurgery, multiple long freezes may be required. Freeze times may need to be increased when treating any cryoresistant lesions.

• *Prolonged ulcer formation was noted after the treatment.* Areas with poor circulation may be susceptible to prolonged ulcer formation. Elderly individuals and patients with diabetes mellitus may be particularly at risk. Certain body locations may also have compromised blood flow, and the skin over the shin, ankle, and foot should be treated cautiously with cryosurgery.

PHYSICIAN TRAINING

Cryosurgery is an easy technique to perform. Most physicians require only 2 to 5 precepted procedures before feeling comfortable performing unassisted procedures. Skill in determining the proper length of freeze, however, can require extensive experience. Physicians in training should begin by per-

TABLE 17.4. CPT Codes for Skin Cryosurgery of Benign or Premalignant Lesions

CPT Codes	Description	1998 Total RVUs[a]	1998 Average 50% Fees in U.S.[b]
17000	Destruction by any method, including laser, with or without surgical curettement; all benign or premalignant lesions other than skin tags or cutaneous vascular proliferative lesions, including local anesthesia; first lesion	1.05	$85
17003	Second through 14th lesions, each (list separately in addition to code for first lesion)	0.29	$23
17004	15 or more lesions	5.24	$419

CPT only © 1998 American Medical Association. All rights reserved.

[a] Department of Health and Human Services, Health Care Financing Administration. Medicare program: revisions to payment policies and adjustments to the relative value units (RVUs) under the physician fee schedule for calendar year 1998. Federal Register 42 CFR part 414. October 31, 1997;62(211):59103–59255.

[b] 1998 Physicians' Fee Reference. West Allis, WI: Yale Wasserman, DMD, Medical Publishers, 1998.

forming cryosurgery on nonfacial lesions before tackling facial lesions, especially in darkly pigmented individuals. Additional formal training is available from the American Academy of Family Physicians.

ORDERING INFORMATION

Gas pressure gauge, cryotips, and cryosurgical administration system (Circon Surgitec, 3037 Mount Pleasant Street, Racine, WI 53404; 800-942-2268)

Nitrous oxide tanks—usually available through local medical supply houses

Water-soluble jelly (K-Y jelly, Johnson & Johnson Medical Inc., 2500 East Arbrook Boulevard, Arlington, TX 76014; 817-645-3141)

BIBLIOGRAPHY

Cryomedics. Guidelines for cryosurgery. Langhorne, PA: Cabot Medical, 1989.

Graham GF. Advances in cryosurgery in the past decade. Cutis 1993;52:365–372.

Grealish RJ. Cryosurgery for benign skin lesions. Family Practice Recertification 1989;11:21–24.

Hocutt JE. Skin cryosurgery for the family physician. Am Fam Physician 1993;48:445–452.

Jones SK, Darville JM. Transmission of virus particles by cryotherapy and multi-use caustic pencils: a problem to dermatologists? Br J Dermatol 1989;121:481–486.

Kuflik EG. Specific indications for cryosurgery of the nail unit: myxoid cysts and periungual verrucae. J Dermatol Surg Oncol 1992;18:702–706.

Torre D. Cutaneous cryosurgery: current state of the art. J Dermatol Surg Oncol 1985;11:292–293.

Torre D. Cryosurgery of basal cell carcinoma. J Am Acad Dermatol 1986;15(pt 1):917–929.

Torre D. The art of cryosurgery. Cutis 1994;54:354.

Zalla MJ. Basic cutaneous surgery [Review]. Cutis 1994;53:172–186.

DIAGNOSTIC AND THERAPEUTIC PROCEDURES

CHAPTER 18
....

Dermal Electrosurgical Shave Excision

Shave excision describes the technique of sharp removal of epidermal or dermal lesions by horizontal slicing. Skin lesions can be removed by electrosurgical technique, conventional scissors, or scalpel shaving methods.

Shave excision usually extends to the level of the middle dermis, with the subcutaneous tissue left undisturbed. The shave biopsy is ideally suited for pedunculated lesions raised above the level of the surrounding skin. Skin lesions with a minimal dermal component, such as seborrheic keratoses or fibrous papules of the nose, are also excellent candidates for shave excision technique.

It is essential when using the shave technique to go deep enough beneath the lesion to remove all the cells of the growth (to prevent recurrence). Generally, the deeper an excision extends into the dermis, the more scarring is produced. Fortunately, most excision sites heal with minimal postoperative scarring and pigmentary changes.

Electrosurgery refers to the cutting and coagulation of tissue using very high-frequency, low-voltage electrical currents. A blended current combines cutting and coagulation, and is useful in producing a bloodless operative field. Lesion excisions on the face are usually performed with only a cutting current to limit scarring at the wound base, which can be produced by thermal coagulation effects. A clear chemical hemostatic agent, such as 85% aluminum chloride, can provide the necessary hemostasis.

Inexperienced physicians often find it easiest to control the depth of excision by using a No. 15 blade held horizontal to the skin surface, which is then brought across the base of the lesion with long, unidirectional strokes.

Electrosurgical feathering (smoothing of the edges using fine brush strokes with the electrode) can then be performed to eliminate sharp wound edges and to contour the wound to the surrounding skin. Feathering is generally performed only with an electrosurgical cutting current.

The dermal electrosurgical shave technique is a fast and inexpensive excision technique that does not require suture closure. This technique is ideally suited for the busy physician, because the setup and procedure can

TABLE 18.1. Lesions Amenable to Shave Excision

Acrochordon (skin tag)
Angiofibroma
Basal cell carcinoma (well-defined, small, low-risk area, primary)
Cutaneous horn
Dermatofibroma
Fibrous papula
Keratoacanthoma
Molluscum contagiosum
Nonpigmented nevi
Papilloma
Rhinophyma
Seborrheic keratosis
Stucco keratoses
Syringoma
Venous lake
Wart

be performed rapidly. Electrosurgical generators on mobile carts can be moved into different examination rooms, thus facilitating the procedure performance in the office setting (Table 18.1).

METHODS AND MATERIALS

Patient Preparation

The patient is seated (or lying) comfortably with the skin lesion exposed.

Equipment

Place the following items on a sterile paper drape over the Mayo stand:

Nonsterile gloves

A 5- or 10-mL syringe filled with 2% lidocaine (Xylocaine) with or without epinephrine, and a 30-gauge needle

No. 15 blade

TABLE 18.2. Lesions Best Considered for Alternative Excision Technique

Pigmented nevi (pathology specimen should be a full thickness skin specimen down to the subcutaneous fat in the event the lesion is a melanoma.)
Skin appendage lesions (syringomas, cylindromas, epidermoid cysts)
Subcutaneous lesions (may be missed by shave technique)

1 inch of 4×4 gauze

A small disposable plastic cup containing povidone-iodine solution

Formalin container

6 small cotton-tipped applicators

A small disposable plastic cup containing Monsel's solution

A small disposable plastic cup containing 85% aluminum chloride (if lesion is on the face)

Electrosurgical Cart

Electrosurgical generator

Smoke evacuator with a special small particle (viral) filtration system

Small dermal loop electrodes

PROCEDURE DESCRIPTION

1. Place the patient in a comfortable seated or lying position with the skin lesion exposed and illuminated. The lesion is prepped with povidone-iodine solution and anesthetized with 2% lidocaine with epinephrine (3-mL syringe with a 30-gauge needle, or a 10-mL syringe if multiple lesions are to be removed). The lesion should be raised with the administration of the anesthetic fluid (Fig. 18.1). Intradermal administration of the fluid creates a blanch to the tissue that indicates the extent of anesthesia. Administer enough fluid to have a ring of anesthesia at least 1 cm from the lesion in all directions.
2. The area can be reprepped with povidone-iodine solution. The initial shave can be performed with a No. 15 blade held in the physician's hand, moving beneath the lesion horizontal to the skin surface. Experienced physicians may chose to remove the lesion with the electrosurgical loop (Fig. 18.2). The specimen is immediately placed in formalin. Bleeding from the wound base is controlled by applying Monsel's solution (ferric subsulfate) or clear 85% aluminum chloride on the face with a cotton swab.
3. The smoke evacuator is turned on, and the assistant holds the tubing next to the site where the electrosurgery is being performed. The smoke evacuator has a special filter, and prevents the dispersion of viral particles such as human immunodeficiency virus (HIV) and human papillomavirus (HPV). Use the smoke evacuator the entire time that electrosurgery is being performed.
4. Electrosurgical feathering is performed with a small dermal loop electrode, using electrosurgical cutting and a setting of 1.5 to 2 (Fig. 18.3). The handpiece is held in the operator's dominant hand, and short strokes (like the strokes of a fine painter) are made with the side of the electrode over the wound edges. The operator's fifth finger rests on the nearby

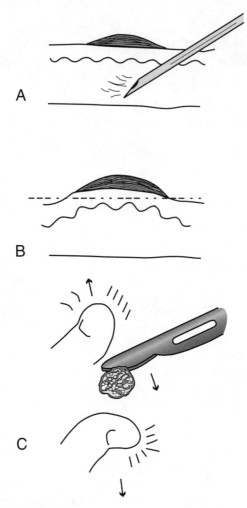

FIGURE 18.1. Shave biopsy technique. The anesthetic is placed below the skin lesion **(A)**, effectively floating the lesion upward **(B)**. The blade is held horizontal to the skin surface and brought below the lesion. The nondominant hand is used to stretch and stabilize the skin surrounding the lesion during the shave biopsy **(C)**. Smooth, unidirectional cutting with the blade separates the lesion above from the deep (reticular) dermis below.

tissues, thus stabilizing the operator's hand. The feathering removes additional cells from the wound base, while smoothing the wound edges and blending the final wound color into the surrounding tissue.

5. Feel with your finger to ensure that no edges remain at the shave site.

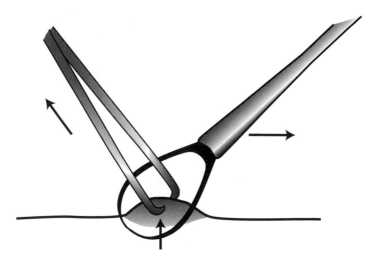

FIGURE 18.2. Electrosurgical loop technique. The lesion is grasped with forceps through the loop electrode, the electrode is activated going under the lesion, and removing the growth.

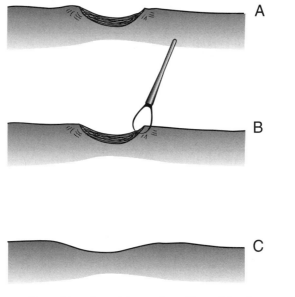

FIGURE 18.3. Smoothing shave biopsy sites. Shave biopsies or excisions can result in circular, crater-like defects that produce a step-off, create shadowing, and can leave a noticeable scar **(A)**. Some surgeons advocate the smoothing of shave biopsy skin edges to blend the healing wound into the surrounding tissues. Electrosurgical cutting using a low power setting can be effectively performed with a thin wire dermal loop **(B)**. The technique of electrosurgical "feathering" uses rapid, short brush strokes to smooth the edges and create a more cosmetically acceptable result **(C)**.

If an edge can be felt, perform additional electrosurgical feathering to smooth the surface.

6. Reapply Monsel's solution if any bleeding persists. Apply an antibiotic ointment, such as Mycitracin Plus, which includes a topical anesthetic. Apply a bandage and give the patient the postprocedure instruction sheet.

FOLLOW UP

* The histologic evaluation of the shave specimen may report a wide variety of benign growths such as angiofibroma, skin tag, or dermatofibroma. If the evaluation of a benign growth reveals that the specimen margin was positive (some cells remained at the excision edge), the lesion can probably be closely followed. Re-excision of the site is generally performed only if regrowth of the tumor is noted at a later date.
* Specimens revealing malignancy with positive margins should prompt consideration for re-excision of the site. Some experts do not recommend automatic re-excision for basal cell carcinomas, because of the superficial nature of these tumors. The electrosurgical shave excision technique also removes additional cells from the wound base, and this may prevent recurrence when the initial shave specimen margin was positive. Several studies have demonstrated that re-excision of basal cell carcinomas with positive margins produces a high frequency of second specimens negative for malignancy. Basal cell carcinomas at low-risk sites, such as the cheek or neck, may be followed closely.
* If a shave excision specimen reveals squamous cell carcinoma, full thickness re-excision of the site is recommended to completely eradicate the potentially metastatic lesion.
* Ideally, a melanoma should never be shaved through, because therapy and long-term prognosis of the malignancy depends on the thickness of the lesion at histologic analysis. If a shaved specimen is reported to contain melanoma, consider specialty referral to a melanoma clinic.
* Occasionally, patients may develop an excessive scar reaction known as a hypertrophic scar. This complication is more common at sites that have excessive tension on the scar, such as over the sternum, over the shoulder, or over flexion creases. Hypertrophic scars often shrink over time, and many experts choose to follow these lesions, or treat them with single or multiple corticosteroid injections.

PROCEDURE PITFALLS/COMPLICATIONS

* *Shaving lesions on the face produces very noticeable scars.* Scars on the face are usually noticeable because wound edges cast a shadow, or because the final white scar is markedly different in color from the surrounding tissue. Electrosurgical feathering smooths sharp wound edges,

and gradually contours and grades the tissue from the wound base to the surrounding tissue. This contouring helps blend the final wound color into the surrounding tissue.

* *The electrosurgical shave went too deep and entered the subcutaneous fat.* The shave technique is an intradermal excision technique. It is rare in family practice to enter the subcutaneous tissue. If the physician unintentionally enters the subcutaneous fat, it is recommended that the procedure be changed to a full thickness excision performed with a sterile surgical tray and a sterile field.

* *The shave technique was used to remove a pigmented nevi.* Shave technique should not be selected for the removal of pigmented lesions that have any potential of being a melanoma. Melanomas can rarely masquerade as a benign pigmented lesion, and a good rule to follow is to remove all pigmented lesions by excision. The prognosis and treatment of melanoma depends on the lesion thickness, and a shave through a melanoma can prevent appropriate histologic identification.

* *Too much tissue is scooped out when excising the lesion with the loop electrode.* Physicians who are inexperienced in the electrosurgical shave technique often remove too much tissue with the first pass of the loop electrode. To limit the scooping effect, some physicians find it easier to control the depth of the initial excision by using a No. 15 blade. The electrosurgical loop is then used to feather the edges, removing additional cells from the wound base and refining the final wound appearance.

* *During the procedure the patient receives an unintentional burn.* The physician must be looking at the electrode tip whenever the electrode is activated. A burn can occur if the electrode is activated while being held close to another part of the patient's skin.

* *The patient complains of pain during the feathering of the wound edges.* Adequate anesthesia should be administered to prevent patient discomfort during the procedure. Electrosurgical feathering extends out from the wound base in all directions. Enough anesthetic should be infiltrated into the skin to produce a blanching that extends at least 1 cm from the lesion edge in all directions.

PHYSICIAN TRAINING

The mechanical techniques of electrosurgical shave excision appear simple, but expertise in creating cosmetically superior wounds can take years to acquire. Electrosurgical feathering can be a very difficult technique to master. Physicians in training should perform as many shave procedures as possible on nonfacial lesions. Once the fine hand motions have been mastered, re-

TABLE 18.3. CPT Codes for Shave Excision

CPT Codes	Description	1998 Total RVUs[a]	1998 Average 50% Fees in U.S.[b]
11300	TAL < 0.5 cm	1.09	$95
11301	TAL 0.6 to 1.0 cm	1.58	$120
11302	TAL 1.1 to 2.0 cm	2.03	$153
11303	TAL > 2.0 cm	2.77	$229
11305	SNHFG < 0.5 cm	1.24	$100
11306	SNHFG 0.6 to 1.0 cm	1.77	$127
11307	SNHFG 1.1 to 2.0 cm	2.18	$178
11308	SNHFG > 2.0 cm	2.98	$276
11310	Face MM < 0.5 cm	1.48	$113
11311	Face MM 0.6 to 1.0 cm	1.98	$158
11312	Face MM 1.1 to 2.0 cm	2.43	$198
11313	Face MM > 2.0 cm	3.26	$300

TAL = trunk, arm, or leg; SNHFG = scalp, neck, hand, foot, or genitalia; face MM = face, ear, eyelid, nose, lip, or mucous membrane.

CPT only © 1998 American Medical Association. All rights reserved.

[a] Department of Health and Human Services, Health Care Financing Administration. Medicare program: revisions to payment policies and adjustments to the relative value units (RVUs) under the physician fee schedule for calendar year 1998. Federal Register 42 CFR part 414. October 31, 1997;62(211):59103–59255.

[b] 1998 Physicians' Fee Reference. West Allis, WI: Yale Wasserman, DMD, Medical Publishers, 1998.

moval of facial excisions can be attempted. It is recommended that physicians receive formal training in electrosurgical currents, such as the courses in electrosurgery offered by the American Academy of Family Physicians.

ORDERING INFORMATION

Aluminum chloride 30%–85%—usually can be obtained from a local pharmacy

Ellman Surgitron electrosurgical unit, electrodes, smoke evacuator (Ellman International, 1135 Railroad Avenue, Hewlett, NY 11557; 800-835-5355)

Formalin CMS Protocol (30-mL bottle; 10% neutral buffered formalin, Biochemical Science, 200 Commodore Drive, Swedesboro, NJ 08085; 800-524-0294)

Povidone-iodine solution 10% (16 fl oz; Povidine, United Research Laboratories, 1100 Orthodox Street, Philadelphia, PA 19124; 215-638-2626)

Xylocaine hydrochloride with epinephrine (50 mL; lidocaine HCl 2% with epinephrine 1:200,000; Astra U.S.A., Inc., 50 Otis Street, Westborough, MA 01581; 508-366-1100)

BIBLIOGRAPHY

Fewkes JL, Sober AJ. Skin biopsy: the four types and how best to do them. Prim Care Cancer 1993;13:36–39.

Habif TP. Clinical dermatology: a color guide to diagnosis and therapy. St Louis: Mosby, 1990.

Hainer BL. Electrosurgery for cutaneous lesions. Am Fam Physician 1991;445(Suppl):81S–90S.

Pariser RJ. Skin biopsy: lesion selection and optimal technique. Modern Med 1989;57:82–90.

Phillips PK, Pariser DM, Pariser RJ. Cosmetic procedures we all perform [Review]. Cutis 1994;53:187–191.

Pollack SV. Electrosurgery of the skin. New York: Churchill Livingstone, 1991.

Stegman SJ, Tromovitch TA, Glogau RG. Basics of dermatologic surgery. Chicago: Year Book Medical Publishers, 1982.

Swanson NA. Atlas of cutaneous surgery. Boston: Little Brown, 1987.

Wyre HW, Stolar R. Extirpation of warts by a loop electrode and cutting current. J Dermatol Surg Oncol 1977;3:520–522.

Zalla MJ. Basic cutaneous surgery [Review]. Cutis 1994;53:172–186.

Zuber TJ. Skin biopsy techniques: when and how to perform shave and excisional biopsy. Consultant 1994;34:1515–1521.

CHAPTER 19

Fine-Needle Aspiration of the Breast

Fine-needle aspiration (FNA) of the breast is a quick, easy, cost-effective technique for evaluating palpable breast lumps. FNA can rapidly distinguish a cystic from solid lesion and can be used to differentiate benign from malignant growths. The technique can be both diagnostic and therapeutic for breast cysts, resulting in symptom reduction and cyst resolution.

Aspiration of breast cysts can yield many different colored fluids. The fluid obtained at cyst aspiration is usually sent for cytologic evaluation only when it is bloody. Non-bloody fluid is almost never associated with an underlying malignancy, and it is not cost-effective to evaluate all aspirated fluid. If a mass persists adjacent to a drained cyst, many experts recommend excision of the mass to exclude a cystic carcinoma.

If fluid is not obtained once the lesion is entered, the solid lesion can be evaluated by passing the needle tip back and forth 20 times within the lesion. FNA of solid lesions has a false-negative rate of 0 to 30%, depending on the experience of the physician performing the aspiration and the pathologist evaluating the slides. The better international centers have false-negative rates of about 4 to 5%. This compares well with mammography, which has about a 4 to 19% average false-negative rate.

Physicians are cautioned not to rely on FNA alone in the evaluation of solid breast lesions. FNA is best used in conjunction with physician examination and mammography, also called the triple diagnostic technique. The triple diagnostic technique yields greater than a 98 to 99% predictive value when all three modalities suggest a lesion is benign; however, a negative cytology does not rule out malignancy, especially when the mammogram or physician's physical examination suggests the presence of malignancy.

FNA can produce hematomas and other artificial changes that can lead to erroneous mammogram interpretation. It is recommended by many experts that the mammogram be performed before or 3 weeks after FNA. Physicians should not fear cancer spread by FNA. Several studies have confirmed that FNA does not spread cancer along the needle tract when it is encountered. In addition, nonpalpable or mammographically detected

169

lesions should not be evaluated by FNA; they are better investigated by stereotactic biopsy. Despite the limitations of FNA, the low cost and decreased invasiveness of the technique make it a useful adjunct in the evaluation of palpable breast masses.

METHODS AND MATERIALS

Patient Preparation

The patient should undress from the waist up and put on a gown. The patient can remain seated on the table to talk with the physiciain. For the procedure, the patient lies supine on the table, with the ipsilateral arm raised above the head.

Equipment

Place the following items on a nonsterile tray:

Nonsterile gloves

4×4 gauze

Alcohol wipes

3 mL syringe with a 30 gauge needle attached filled with 2% lidocaine with epinephrine (Xylocaine with epinephrine), if desired

2 Euro-Med FNA 21 needles (one is for backup if an additional aspiration is performed)

4 glass slides with patient name and date written on the frosted end of the slides

Transport container for the slides (for transport to the laboratory)

Cytofixative spray

Bandage

PROCEDURE DESCRIPTION

1. The patient undresses from the waist up and puts on a gown. The patient is placed supine on the table, and the ipsilateral arm raised above the head. The breast lump is isolated using the fingers of the nondominant hand. Often the lump can be surrounded by the fingertips and lifted up toward the skin. The lump should be held tightly enough to prevent movement. It is recommended that the physician wear nonsterile gloves, although sometimes the glove of the nondominant hand must be removed if it interferes with the ability to feel the lump.

2. The skin is cleansed with an alcohol swab. Some physicians prefer to anesthetize the skin overlying the lump using 2% lidocaine with epinephrine. Others believe that the needle insertion for anesthesia causes as much

discomfort as the aspiration itself and choose to perform the procedure without anesthesia.

3. The needle tip is inserted into the mass, with the fingertips of the nondominant hand confirming that the tip is in the proper place (Fig. 19.1). Negative pressure is applied in the syringe, producing a vacuum effect. Cysts will drain readily. If the fluid is bloody, it is sent to the laboratory for cytologic assessment. A solid lesion is evaluated by collecting microfragments shaved off from repetitive passes back and forth within the lesion. The needle tip should be moved up and down 20 times, keeping the tip within the lump. The excursion of the needle depends on the size of the lump, as the tip can remain in a small lump only with a small amount of movement. The fragments of tissue will be pulled up into the hub of the syringe.

4. Once an adequate tissue sample is in the needle and syringe hub, the pressure on the syringe is released. The needle is withdrawn from the skin. Gauze is applied over the aspiration site, and the nurse or patient holds direct pressure over the aspiration site for 5 minutes. A bandage is then applied.

5. The cellular contents in the needle and hub are gently expressed onto one or two glass slides (Fig. 19.2). Usually a single drop of material is expressed onto each slide. A clean slide then is pressed upside down onto the slide containing the cellular material. The two slides are gently slid in opposite directions, smearing the cellular material uniformly over both of the slides. Each slide is sprayed immediately with cytofixative spray, and sent for cytologic assessment. This technique yields two to four slides for each site aspirated.

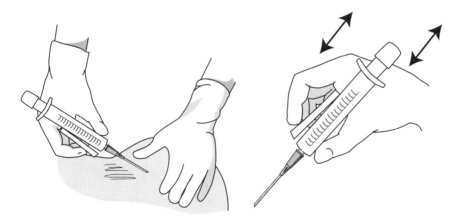

FIGURE 19.1.   The breast mass is stabilized using the nondominant hand. The needle is inserted into the lesion and, if the mass is solid, then 20 passes are made with an up and down motion, keeping the needle tip within the lesion.

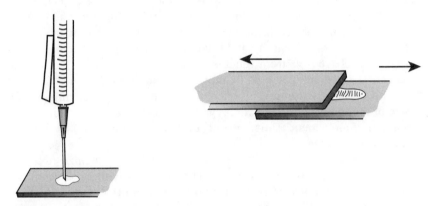

FIGURE 19.2. The material in the hub of the syringe is gently expressed onto a slide, and a second slide is placed on top of the first. The two slides are gently pulled in opposite directions, causing the material to be evenly smeared, and the slides are immediately sprayed with fixative.

FOLLOW UP

- Aspiration frequently yields brown, black, yellow, or greenish serous fluid. It is not cost-effective to evaluate all aspirated fluid. Most experts recommend sending only bloody aspirated fluid for cytology examination. Non-bloody fluid is almost never associated with an underlying malignancy.
- If a mass persists after fluid is aspirated from a cyst, excision of the mass is recommended to exclude malignancy.
- Patients should be reexamined 1 month after breast cyst aspiration. If the cyst has redeveloped, re-aspiration is recommended. If the cyst reforms after a second aspiration, then excision of the cyst is recommended to exclude malignancy.
- Follow up of patients after aspiration of cellular material from a solid breast lesion is outlined in Table 19.1.

PROCEDURE PITFALLS/COMPLICATIONS

- *The patient becomes dyspneic after needle aspiration (pneumothorax).* Pneumothorax has been documented after breast needle aspiration. This unusual complication develops when the needle is placed too deep, with the needle tip penetrating the pleural space. Caution during the needle insertion, especially into a small breast, can reduce the incidence of this complication. The patient should be followed clinically and radio-graphically, and hospitalized if symptomatic.

- *Bleeding in the breast after the procedure.* The needle can cause bleeding from the highly vascular skin or breast tissue. As the needle is withdrawn at the end of the procedure, immediate direct pressure is applied for 5 minutes with gauze over the aspiration site. If excess bleeding is noted during the aspiration, the patient can continue direct pressure for 10-20 more minutes to reduce bruising in the breast tissue.

- *The aspiration attempt fails to sample the palpable lump.* It is possible to miss sampling the palpable lump by placing the needle tip above, below, or to the side of the lesion. This error can be minimized by isolating the lump in the fingertips of the nondominant hand. By stabilizing and elevating the lesion, the proper depth can be confirmed when the needle tip enters the lesion.

- *The pathologist reports the sample is an acellular aspiration or is unsatisfactory due to limited cellularity.* Correct technique occasionally produces an acellular or limited cellular specimen. Acellular smears should not compromise more than about 10 to 20% of all the reports generated for breast aspirations. If enough passes are made with the needle tip within the lesion, some cellularity should be obtained in the majority of the procedures.

TABLE 19.1. Breast Needle Aspiration Cytology of Solid Lesions and Suggested Follow Up

Result	Suggested Follow Up
Scant/insufficient cells for diagnosis	Repeat needle aspiration, or biopsy if clinical suspicion is high
Benign—fibroadenoma	Reassurance or symptomatic treatment, if cellular changes are not complex or associated with atypical hyperplasia
Benign—fibrocystic	Symptomatic treatment, if not associated with atypical hyperplasia
Benign—other (includes fat necrosis, lipoma, inflammation, papilloma, and other benign ductal epithelium)	Reassurance and clinical follow-up
Atypical cells	Clinical follow-up only if reactive or degenerative atypia (seen in fibrocystic change); mammogram and biopsy if severe atypia
Suspicion of malignancy	Surgical referral and biopsy
Malignant cells	Surgical referral and biopsy

• *A cyst continues to refill after two separate needle aspirations.* It is recommended that the breast should be reexamined 1 month after cyst drainage. If the cyst refills, the lesion can be re-aspirated. If the cyst refills after the second procedure, then excision is recommended to exclude a cystic carcinoma adjacent to the site.

• *Patient develops cancer following a negative aspiration.* Fine-needle aspiration of the breast has a significant false-negative rate. It is best used in conjunction with mammography and physician examination. This triple diagnostic technique yields a 98–99% predictive value when all three modalities suggest a lesion is benign. If any of the three suggest malignancy, further evaluation is warranted.

PHYSICIAN TRAINING

Breast needle aspiration is an easy procedure to perform. Stabilizing the mass in the nondominant hand and keeping the needle tip within the mass while moving the needle back and forth are the two most difficult techniques to master. Most residency-trained physicians are skilled in other needle techniques (blood drawing, injections, etc.) and can perform breast needle aspiration after just a few precepted procedures.

ORDERING INFORMATION

Cameco syringe pistol (handle for holding disposable Becton-Dickinson 10-mL syringes and disposable 21-gauge needles; Precision Dynamics Corporation, 13880 Del Sur Street, San Fernando, CA 91340; 800-847-0670; one-time cost about $250)

TABLE 19.2. CPT Codes

CPT Codes	Description	1998 Total RVUs[a]	1998 Average 50% Fees in U.S.[b]
19000	Puncture aspiration of cyst of breast	1.29	$107
19001	Cyst aspiration, each additional	0.71	$63
88170	Fine-needle aspiration, breast lesion with or without preparation of smears; superficial tissue	—	$94

CPT only © 1998 American Medical Association. All rights reserved.

[a] Department of Health and Human Services, Health Care Financing Administration. Medicare program: revisions to payment policies and adjustments to the relative value units (RVUs) under the physician fee schedule for calendar year 1998. Federal Register 42 CFR part 414. October 31, 1997;62(211):59103–59255.

[b] 1998 Physicians' Fee Reference. West Allis, WI: Yale Wasserman, DMD, Medical Publishers, 1998.

Cytofixative (CMS Protocol cytologic fixative; Biochemical Science, 200 Commodore Drive, Swedesboro, NJ 08085; 800-524-0294)

Disposable FNA 21 needle (Euro-Med, Cooper Surgical, 15 Forest Parkway, Shelton, CT 06484; 800-848-0033; about $10 per disposable spring-loaded syringe and 21-gauge needle)

BIBLIOGRAPHY

Connolly DP. Fine-needle aspiration of the breast. Family Practice Recertification 1992;14:32-37.

Cowen PN, Benson EA. Cytological study of fluid from breast cysts. Br J Surg 1979;66:209-211.

Erickson R, Shank JC, Gratton C. Fine-needle breast aspiration biopsy. J Fam Pract 1989;28:306-309.

Frable WJ. Thin-needle aspiration biopsy: a personal experience with 469 cases [Review]. Am J Clin Pathol 1976;65:168-182.

Frable WJ. Needle aspiration biopsy: past, present, and future. Hum Pathol 1989;20:504-517.

Kline TS. Fine-needle aspiration biopsy of the breast. Am Fam Physician 1995;52:2021-2025.

Layfield LJ, Chrischilles EA, Cohen MB, Bottles K. The palpable breast nodule: a cost-effectiveness analysis of alternate diagnostic approaches. Cancer 1993;72:1642-1651.

Place R, Velanovich V, Carter P. Fine needle aspiration in the clinical management of mammary masses. Surg Gynecol Obstet 1993;177:7-11.

Waisman J. Diagnostic aspiration of palpable mammary lesions. Prim Care Cancer 1992;12:31-36.

Wollenberg NJ, Caya LG, Clowry LJ. Fine needle aspiration cytology of the breast: a review of 321 cases with statistical evaluation. Acta Cytol 1985;29:425-429.

CHAPTER 20

Fusiform Excision

The fusiform excision technique is commonly used by family physicians for removing skin and subcutaneous lesions. This office procedure offers the advantages of a definitive, single-stage diagnostic and therapeutic intervention. The fusiform excision has previously been referred to as an elliptical excision, but the true biconcave appearance of the wound is more appropriately described as fusiform. Shave excision is a more simple procedure, but the fusiform excision technique offers cosmetic and diagnostic advantage for certain clinical situations. The fusiform technique should be used to biopsy any pigmented lesions that potentially could be a melanoma, because the future therapy of a melanoma is dependent on the depth of the lesion.

The classical fusiform excision has a 3 : 1 length-to-width ratio. This technique produces an angle of 30 degrees or less at the end of the wound. The long axis of the wound should be oriented parallel to the lines of least skin tension in order to improve the final scar outcome. A properly designed fusiform excision can be closed primarily and should not result in the formation of raised tissue at the ends of the wound (known as dog-ears).

Gentle handling of the wound edges with skin hooks produces good cosmetic results. The skin should not be grasped with forceps, because the resulting skin damage can produce necrosis and scarring. Disposable skin hooks can be created by bending the end of a 21-gauge needle. Disposable skin hooks are preferred by nursing personnel, because accidents in the process of autoclaving frequently occur when skin hooks break through the sterile wraps.

Hematomas at the base of an excision inhibit wound healing, create excessive scarring and produce a depressed and more noticeable scar following normal scar retraction. Subcutaneous bleeding sites can be controlled with instrument clamps, electrocautery or absorbable suture ligation. Interrupted, deep-buried absorbable sutures placed down to the level of the fascia eliminate dead space, provide excellent hemostasis, reduce tension on the skin sutures, and generally improve the cosmetic and functional result.

METHODS AND MATERIALS

Patient Preparation

The patient is seated or lying comfortably with the skin lesion exposed.

Equipment

Nonsterile Tray for Anesthesia and Designing the Fusiform Excision

  Nonsterile gloves

  Skin marking pen

  4 × 4 gauze

  Povidone-iodine solution

  1 10-mL syringe with a 30-gauge needle attached, filled with 1% lidocaine
    with epinephrine (Xylocaine with epinephrine)

  Mask

Sterile Tray for the Procedure

Place the following items on a sterile disposable drape covering a Mayo stand:

  Sterile gloves

  Fenestrated disposable drape

  Additional nonfenestrated disposable drape (if desired)

  2 sterile bandages to anchor the fenestrated drape

  3 hemostats (Mosquito clamps)

  No. 15 scalpel blade and handle

  Needle holder

  Mayo or tissue scissors

  Iris scissors for cutting sutures

  Adson forceps

  21-gauge, 1 ½-inch needle (to be bent into a skin hook)

  2 inches of 4×4 gauze

  Suture materials

PROCEDURE DESCRIPTION

1. The fusiform excision is designed with a 3 : 1 length-to-width ratio, oriented in the direction of the lines of least skin tension (Figs. 20.1 and 20.2).
   The excision lines can be marked on the skin using a skin marking pen.
2. The skin is prepped with povidone-iodine solution, and the skin is anesthetized with 1% or 2% lidocaine with or without epinephrine. The hemostatic benefit of epinephrine is added for most procedures, except when

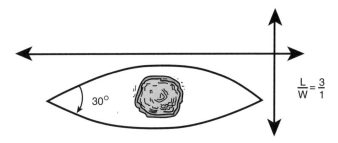

$$\frac{L}{W} = \frac{3}{1}$$

30°

FIGURE 20.1. A properly designed fusiform excision has a length-to-width ratio of 3 to 1. In addition, the angle at the corner of the fusiform island of tissue should be 30° or less.

the surgery is performed on the digits or the tip of the nose. The anesthetic can be administered with a 30-gauge needle attached to a 10-mL syringe, for enhanced patient comfort.

3. Following administration of the anesthetic, sterile gloves can be applied, the skin can be reprepped with povidone-iodine solution, and a sterile fenestrated paper drape placed over the surgical field. Sterile bandages can be used at the edge of the fenestration to keep the drape from shifting and prevent unprepped skin from appearing through the drape hole.

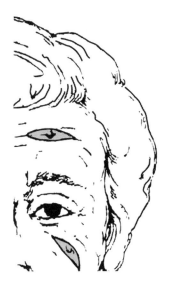

FIGURE 20.2. Fusiform excisions are designed to follow the lines of least skin tension. The lines of least skin tension are influenced by the contractions of the underlying muscles, and they tend to follow skin creases and wrinkles.

4. The incision is made with a No. 15 scalpel blade held vertical to the skin. Inward beveling or "wedging" is discouraged. The first pass of the scalpel on each wound edge should be smooth and continuous to prevent notching of the skin. A second pass of the blade may be needed to extend these incisions down to the level of the fat. Some 4×4 gauze can be used to wipe the surgical field clear of blood.

5. The scalpel is turned parallel to the skin surface to undermine the central fusiform island of skin. The central island of skin is lifted with Adson forceps with teeth as the scalpel is moved in the level of the upper fat. Once the central island of skin is removed, it is immediately placed in formalin for histologic evaluation.

6. Bleeding sites in the wound base can be controlled by applying hemostats or suture ligation. The physician should not be overly preoccupied with bleeding, and should continue efforts to prepare the wound for closure. The lateral tissues are elevated with a skin hook or disposable hook (created by curling the end of a 21-gauge 1 ½ inch needle). The lateral skin edges are not lifted with Adson forceps, because the forceps may cause tissue necrosis. The lateral skin edges are undermined with horizontally held scalpel or scissors, in the level of the upper fat; 3 cm of lateral undermining is required for every 1 cm of skin edge relaxation.

7. Interrupted, deep, buried sutures are placed to eliminate dead space at the wound base, promote healing, reduce tension on the skin sutures, and improve the final cosmetic appearance of the scar (Fig. 20.3). Vicryl sutures (3-0, 4-0, or 5-0) are the most commonly selected absorbable sutures for closure in the office setting. Proper placement of these sutures produces close approximation of the skin edges.

8. The skin edges should be everted (upward lifting of the skin edges) to improve the final scar appearance. Interrupted nylon sutures (4-0, 5-0, or 6-0) are the most commonly selected nonabsorbable sutures for skin closure in the office setting. Eversion often can be accomplished without grasping the skin edges with forceps, by entering and exiting the skin vertically with the suture needle, while depressing lateral tissue with a finger of the nondominant hand.

9. Once the suturing is completed, the wound should be squeezed gently to remove any residual blood from beneath the wound that will interfere with healing. Direct pressure can be applied with gauze by the patient for 5 to 10 minutes to assist with hemostasis. The nurse then cleans the site with saline, applies antibiotic ointment, and places a pressure dressing (Elastoplast over gauze).

FOLLOW UP

• Malignant growths may require a second procedure to provide a wider margin of excision around the original lesion. For instance, a melanoma-

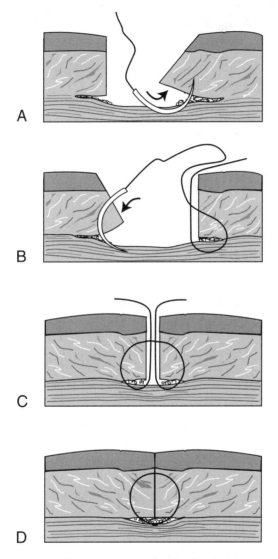

FIGURE 20.3.   Buried knots are created with absorbable subcuticular sutures by taking the first bite on the far side of the wound from bottom to top **(A)**. The bite includes tissue at the base of the wound to close the deep space. The needle is then placed in the needle holder upside down and backwards and a reverse bite is created going from top to bottom on the near side **(B)**. Both the free end of the suture and the needle end must exit the wound on the same side of the suture across the tope of the wound **(C)**. This allows the final knot to be buried in the wound base **(D)**.

TABLE 20.1. Timing of Suture Removal

Facial sutures	3 to 5 days
Scalp and neck sutures	7 days
Upper extremity sutures	7 to 9 days
Upper extremity over a joint crease sutures	8 to 14 days
Trunk sutures	8 to 12 days
Lower extremity sutures	14 to 28 days

in-situ should have a 0.5 cm margin of normal skin removed surrounding the lesion. A thicker melanoma may require a 3 cm margin of normal skin removed in all directions around the lesion.

- Malignancies that are not completely excised at the original biopsy may require re-excision. When the pathologist reports positive margins, consideration should be given to a second procedure. Basal cell carcinomas that infiltrate through the skin, such as the morpheaform type, may not have visible margins and may require Mohs' surgery or wide excision for complete removal. Squamous cell carcinomas that have positive margins at the original excision should be removed with an excision of the suture line and surrounding tissue on the sides and below the original surgical site.

- Some pathology reports may describe rare or unusual tumors that are unfamiliar to the family physician. Pathologists may also use ambiguous terminology in describing a lesion. If there is confusion or uncertainty, speak directly to the pathologist. Many pathologists welcome the clinical interchange with the physician. Patients can be referred to more experienced surgeons for unfamiliar findings or uncertain management.

- Skin suture removal should be performed in an appropriate interval following the original surgery. Many factors influence the timing of suture removal, including the patient's age, nutritional status, and other medical problems, such as diabetes. A general guide for suture removal based on the body site is listed in Table 20.1.

- Patients may be upset if their wound undergoes dehiscence. Physicians should be careful when early suture removal is attempted, especially on the lower extremity. Surgical wounds generally have only 8 to 15% of their final wound strength two weeks following the procedure. At the time of suture removal, consider applying tincture of benzoin solution to the skin and steri-strips to provide additional wound strength for an additional seven to 10 days.

PROCEDURE PITFALLS/COMPLICATIONS

- *Excessive bleeding occurred during the procedure.* Excision of the fusiform island of skin and lateral edge undermining can produce vigorous bleeding, which can sidetrack inexperienced physicians. Avoid wasting time in repetitive blotting of the wound bed with gauze. Learn to work around the bleeding. Bleeding vessels in the wound base can be briefly clamped with hemostats while undermining is performed. Placing the deep, buried, absorbable sutures to approximate skin edges and closing the dead space almost always stops wound bleeding.

- *The wound only closes in the center with hard tugging on the tissues.* Novice physicians often fail to undermine the lateral tissues adequately. Each skin edge must be undermined 3 cm for every 1 cm gained in tissue relaxation. Extensive undermining does produce some bleeding, but the bleeding is easily controlled with placement of the deep sutures. Failure to perform adequate undermining can cause excessive tension on the center of the wound and subsequent skin breakdown or suture tension marks.

- *Wound infection occurred following the procedure.* Wound infections are uncommon if proper aseptic technique is performed. The operative time should be as short as possible. Antibiotic ointment applied to the wound immediately following the surgery and then daily until the sutures are removed can aid in wound healing and infection prevention. Wound-edge redness that is within ½ inch of the wound and not associated with pus or drainage often is not infection, but reparative or inflammatory changes associated with healing. Care must be taken when performing procedures in certain high-risk areas for infection, such as the groin or lower legs.

- *The wounds frequently have dog-ears at the ends.* Dog-ears are mounds of elevated tissue that occur at the ends of some linear wounds after closure. Dog-ears can occur with excisions on convex surfaces such as the arms and legs. Dog-ears most commonly develop from an improperly designed fusiform excision. The wound should be long enough to have at least a 3 : 1 length-to-width ratio. Dog-ears can be removed by excising a fusiform island of skin in the direction of the original wound or by removing a lateral piece of redundant skin and extending the wound laterally.

- *A seroma developed beneath the wound.* Failure to close the dead space beneath a wound can result in the formation of a seroma (thin-walled pseudocysts that represent collections of serous fluid in an open space). The placement of deep, buried sutures generally eliminates this complication.

- *The excision damaged nerves or arteries beneath the wound.* Incisions that extend deep into tissues have the potential to cause permanent nerve and artery damage. Placing a generous volume of anesthetic beneath a lesion effectively increases the thickness of the skin and subcutaneous tissues, thereby keeping the incisions more superficial. The anesthetic also displaces downward structures in the deep fat, such as arteries and nerves. Undermining the wound edges in the level of the upper fat also helps to avoid damaging deeper structures.

• *The patient experiences discomfort during the procedure.* Novice physicians often do not adequately anesthetize the wound before starting the procedure. Five to 10 mL of anesthetic should be administered before most procedures. The sides of the wound must be infiltrated to provide coverage for the lateral undermining. Intradermal blanching produced by anesthetic administration can be a useful indication that the incision lines are ready for the procedure.

• *The final scar is thick and unsightly.* Properly designed incisions that follow the lines of least-skin tension usually result in cosmetically acceptable scars. Wounds that cross flexion creases or are perpendicular to the lines of least tension can thicken into hypertrophic scars. Physicians may need to consult reference diagrams that describe the orientation of skin tension lines in complex areas (e.g., the face).

• *The final scar has cross-hatch or railroad marks.* Cross-hatching of the final scar often results from too much tension on the wound from the skin sutures. Placing deep subcutaneous sutures can reduce tension on the wound. Placing smaller caliber skin sutures (5-0 and 6-0) closer to the wound edge can reduce the tension across the wound and reduce the formation of cross-hatch marks. The sutures should not be tied too tightly.

TABLE 20.2.   CPT Codes

CPT Codes[a]	Description	1998 Total RVUs[b]	1998 Average 50% Fees in U.S.[c]
11400–11446	Excision, benign lesion	1.49–6.45	$124–$594
11600–11646	Excision, malignant lesion	2.64–10.87	$196–$949
12031–12057	Layer closure of wounds	2.94–12.01	$165–$899

CPT only © 1998 American Medical Association. All rights reserved.

[a] Physicians can select the appropriate CPT code based on whether the lesion is benign or malignant. Malignant excisions reimburse more than benign excisions. Since the pathologist determines the malignant nature of the lesion, the billing can be delayed until the pathology report is available. Physicians may choose to report an intermediate repair, in addition to the excision codes, if a layered repair is needed to close the wound. The excision codes include only a simple (one-layer) repair. In 1997, Medicare defines an intermediate repair as one requiring closure of one or more of the deeper fascial layers, not one that requires layered closure.

[b] Department of Health and Human Services, Health Care Financing Administration. Medicare program: revisions to payment policies and adjustments to the relative value units (RVUs) under the physician fee schedule for calendar year 1998. Federal Register 42 CFR part 414. October 31, 1997;62(211):59103–59255.

[c] 1998 Physicians' Fee Reference. West Allis, WI: Yale Wasserman, DMD, Medical Publishers, 1998.

PHYSICIAN TRAINING

Formal training is needed for the techniques of anesthetic administration, lesion excision, and closure techniques. Most family physicians receive this training in their residency programs. Others can obtain this training with an experienced preceptor. Physicians experienced in skin surgery can often perform these excisions unsupervised after two to five procedures. Inexperienced physicians may require 20 to 40 precepted procedures before attempting unsupervised excisions.

BIBLIOGRAPHY

Borges AF, Alexander JE. Relaxed skin tension lines, Z-plasties on scars, and fusiform excision of lesions. Br J Plast Surg 1962;15:242-254.

Borges AF. Dog-ear repair. Plast Reconstr Surg 1982;69:707-713.

Pories WJ. Biopsies and excision of lesions. In: Pories WJ, Thomas FT, eds. Office surgery for family physicians. Boston: Butterworth, 1985:57-64.

Snyder CC. Scalp, face, and salivary glands. In: Ferguson LK. Ferguson's surgery of the ambulatory patient. 5th ed. Philadelphia: JB Lippincott, 1974:153-181.

Stegman SJ, Tromovitch TA, Glogau RG. Basics of dermatologic surgery. Chicago: Year Book Medical Publishers, 1982.

Stevenson TR, Jurkiewicz MJ. Plastic and reconstructive surgery. In: Schwartz SI, Shires GT, Spencer FC, Husser WC, eds. Principles of surgery. 5th ed. New York: McGraw-Hill, 1989:2081-2132.

Swanson NA. Atlas of cutaneous surgery. Boston: Little Brown, 1987.

Vistnes LM. Basic principles of cutaneous surgery. In: Epstein E, Epstein E Jr, eds. Skin surgery. 6th ed. Philadelphia: WB Saunders, 1987:44-55.

Zitelli J. TIPS for a better ellipse. J Am Acad Dermatol 1990;22:101-103.

Zuber TJ, DeWitt DE. The fusiform excision. Am Fam Physician 1994;49:371-376, 379-380.

CHAPTER 21

Knee Joint Aspiration and Injection

Knee joint aspiration and injection are performed to establish a diagnosis, relieve discomfort, drain off infected fluid, or to instill medication. Because prompt treatment of a joint infection can preserve the joint integrity, any unexplained monarthritis should be considered for arthrocentesis (Table 21.1).

Arthrocentesis also may help to distinguish the inflammatory arthropathies from the crystal arthritides or osteoarthritis. If a hemarthrosis is discovered after trauma, it can indicate the presence of a fracture or other anatomic disruption.

The knee is the most common and easiest joint for the physician to aspirate, and was chosen for discussion here because of the frequent clinical problems associated with this joint. The indications, complications, and pitfalls for knee arthrocentesis generally can be applied to other joints (Tables 21.2 and 21.3). Many of the principles of needle aspiration and injection also can be used for soft tissue disorders, such as bursitis or tendinitis.

An effusion of the knee often produces detectable suprapatellar or parapatellar swelling. Large effusions can produce ballotment of the patella. Medial or lateral approaches to the knee can be selected; some investigators advocate the medial approach when the effusion is small, and the lateral approach with larger effusions. The knee generally is easiest to aspirate when the patient is supine and the knee is extended.

Corticosteroids are believed to modify the vascular inflammatory response to injury, inhibit destructive enzymes, and restrict the action of inflammatory cells. Intrasynovial steroid administration is designed to maximize local benefits and to minimize systemic adverse effects. Local corticosteroid injections can provide significant relief, and often ameliorate acute exacerbations of knee osteoarthritis associated with significant effusions.

There is no convincing evidence that corticosteroids modify rheumatic joint destruction, and steroid injections in patients with rheumatoid arthritis should be considered ancillary to rest, physical therapy, nonsteroidal anti-inflammatory drugs (NSAIDs), or disease-modifying antirheumatic drugs.

Judicious use of corticosteroids rarely produces significant adverse effects. The introduction of infection after injection is believed to occur in less than 1 in 10,000 procedures. The concept of steroid arthropathy is largely based on studies in subprimate animal models, and this is an unusual occurrence in humans if the number of injections is limited to three to four per year in weight-bearing joints. More conservative researchers have even advocated limiting knee injections to three or four over an individual's lifetime.

TABLE 21.1. Indications for Arthrocentesis

Crystal-induced arthropathy
Hemarthrosis
Limiting joint damage from an infectious process
Symptomatic relief of a large effusion
Unexplained joint effusion
Unexplained monarthritis

TABLE 21.2. Contraindications to Intra-Articular Injection

Adjacent osteomyelitis
Bacteremia
Hemarthrosis
Impending (scheduled within days) joint replacement surgery
Infectious arthritis
Joint prosthesis
Osteochondral fracture
Periarticular cellulitis
Poorly controlled diabetes mellitus
Uncontrolled bleeding disorder or coagulopathy

TABLE 21.3. Contraindications to Joint Needle Aspiration

Bacteremia
Clinician unfamiliar with the anatomy or approach to the joint
Inaccessible joints
Joint prosthesis
Overlying infection in the soft tissues
Severe coagulopathy
Severe overlying dermatitis
Uncooperative patient

METHODS AND MATERIALS

Patient Preparation

Clothing is removed from over the affected joint. The patient is placed in the supine position and the knee is extended (some physicians prefer to have the knee bent to 90°). An absorbent pad is placed beneath the knee.

Equipment

Sterile Tray for the Procedure

Place the following items on a sterile sheet covering the Mayo stand:

Sterile gloves

Sterile fenestrated drape

2 10-mL syringes

2 21-gauge 1-inch needles

1 inch of 4×4 gauze soaked with povidone-iodine solution

Hemostat (for stabilizing the needle when exchanging the medication syringe for the aspiration syringe)

Sterile bandage

PROCEDURE DESCRIPTION

1. The patient is supine on the table with the knee extended (some physicians prefer for the knee to be bent to 90°). Some physicians prefer the medial approach for smaller effusions, but the lateral approach will be discussed here. The knee is examined to determine the amount of joint fluid present and to check for overlying cellulitis or coexisting pathology in the joint or surrounding tissues.
2. The superior lateral aspect of the patella is palpated. The skin is marked with a pen, one finger-breadth above and one finger-breadth lateral to this site. This location provides the most direct access to the synovium.
3. The skin is washed with povidone-iodine solution. The physician should be gloved, although there is no consensus as to whether sterile gloves must be used. A 20-gauge 1-inch needle is attached to a 5- to 20-mL syringe, depending on the anticipated amount of fluid present for removal.
4. The needle is inserted through stretched skin. Some physicians administer lidocaine into the skin, but stretching the pain fibers in the skin with the nondominant hand can also reduce needle insertion discomfort. The needle is directed at a 45° angle distally and 45° into the knee, tilted below the patella (Figs. 21.1 and 21.2).

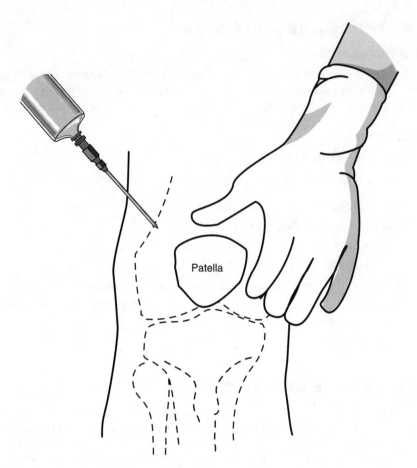

FIGURE 21.1. The technique described involves insertion of the needle 1 cm above and 1 cm lateral to the superior lateral aspect of the patella. The needle is tilted beneath the patella at a 45° angle.

5. Once the needle has been inserted 1 to 1½ inches, aspiration is performed and the syringe should fill with fluid. Using the nondominant hand to compress the opposite side of the joint or the patella may aid in arthrocentesis.

6. Once the syringe has filled, a hemostat can be placed onto the hub of the needle. With the needle stabilized with the hemostat, the syringe can be disconnected and the fluid sent for studies. Be careful not to touch the needle tip against the joint surfaces when removing the syringe. A syringe filled with corticosteroid medication can then be attached to the needle.

7. For injection, use betamethasone (Celestone 6 mg/mL), 1 mL, mixed with

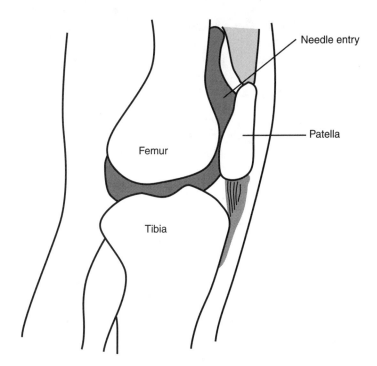

FIGURE 21.2.   The lateral view shows the needle insertion site beneath the patella.

3 to 5 mL of 1% lidocaine. Alternately, methylprednisolone (Depo-Medrol 40 mg/mL), 1 mL, mixed with 3 to 5 mL of 1% lidocaine can be used. After injection of the medication, the needle and syringe are withdrawn.

8. The skin is cleansed and a bandage applied over the needle-puncture site. The patient is warned to avoid forceful activity on the joint while it is anesthetized.

FOLLOW UP

- After diagnostic arthrocentesis, appropriate intervention usually will be dictated by the results of the fluid analysis. Joint infections are usually treated aggressively with intravenous antibiotics. An inflammatory arthritis, such as rheumatoid arthritis, can be treated with disease-modifying medications, such as methotrexate, or penicillamine. Traumatic or bloody effusions may be considered for further orthopedic evaluation.
- Large effusions can recur, and may require repeat aspiration. Anti-inflammatory medications may prove beneficial in reducing joint inflammation and fluid accumulations.

- Corticosteroid injections for osteoarthritis often provide a short-lived benefit. Repeat injections can be considered after 6 weeks. Large, weight-bearing joints should not be injected more than three times a year.

PROCEDURE PITFALLS/COMPLICATIONS

- *The patient complains of severe pain during the procedure.* Severe pain experienced during the procedure usually results from the needle coming into contact with the highly innervated cartilaginous surfaces. The needle can be redirected or withdrawn when pain is encountered. Slow, steady movement of the needle during insertion can prevent damage to the cartilage surface from the needle bevel.

- *The patient's effusion was sterile, but became infected after the joint injection.* Introduction of infection into a joint is a rare event, occurring in less than 0.01% of injections; however, infection can develop when the needle is introduced into the joint through an area of cellulitis. Severe dermatitis or soft tissue infection overlying a joint is a contraindication of arthrocentesis. Some physicians advocate that steroid injection should not be performed before excluding joint infection.

- *The patient complains that the joint hurts much worse the day after the injection than it did before the injection.* A recognized complication of steroid injections to joints is the postinjection flare. The flare reaction represents an increase in joint pain occurring in 1 to 2% of individuals. The steroid crystals can induce an inflammatory synovitis that usually begins about 6 to 12 hours after the injection. The postinjection flare can present with swelling, tenderness, and warmth over the joint that persists for hours to days. If the patient takes anti-inflammatory medications immediately after the injection, then it may reduce or abort this reaction. Aspiration should be performed to rule out joint sepsis if symptoms persist beyond 2 to 3 days.

- *The patient develops joint instability from repeated injections.* The most serious complication of repeated injections is joint instability from the development of osteonecrosis of juxta-articular bone and weakened capsular ligaments. Although this complication occurs in less than 1% of patients, it is recommended that injections be performed no more frequently than every 6 to 8 weeks, and no more than three times per year for weight-bearing joints.

- *A large knee effusion re-accumulated right after being drained.* Large effusions from the knee can rapidly re-accumulate. Some physicians advocate placing an elastic wrap around the knee immediately after large effusion drainage.

- *The patient's pain returned just a few weeks after the injection.* A major disadvantage to intra-articular corticosteroid injections is the short duration of action. The average duration of the injection's benefit may only be 2 to 3 weeks; however, a small percentage of patients with osteoarthritis may have sustained relief after one or two injections.

TABLE 21.4. Arthrocentesis Codes

CPT Codes	Description	1998 Total RVUs[a]	1998 Average 50% Fees in U.S.[b]
20600	Aspiration/injection small joint or bursa (e.g., fingers, toes)	1.18	$69
20605	Aspiration/injection intermediate joint or bursa (e.g., ankle, elbow)	1.18	$75
20610	Aspiration/injection major joint or bursa (e.g., shoulder, knee)	1.29	$86

CPT only © 1998 American Medical Association. All rights reserved.
[a] Department of Health and Human Services, Health Care Financing Administration. Medicare program: revisions to payment policies and adjustments to the relative value units (RVUs) under the physician fee schedule for calendar year 1998. Federal Register 42 CFR part 414. October 31, 1997;62(211):59103–59255.
[b] 1998 Physicians' Fee Reference. West Allis, WI: Yale Wasserman, DMD, Medical Publishers, 1998.

PHYSICIAN TRAINING

Experience is important for the proper performance of joint aspiration and injection procedures. Physicians skilled in arthrocentesis usually have had the opportunity to gain experience with a rheumatologist or other physician who performs many procedures. Each joint has different anatomic landmarks, and novice physicians may need to review a textbook for approaches to an unfamiliar joint. Although arthrocentesis is a simple technique with minimal risk, physicians should have assistance or supervision with their first few attempts at any site. Family physicians wanting to perform arthrocentesis on deep joints, such as the hip or vertebral joints, should obtain extensive training in these higher risk procedures. Additional training in arthrocentesis is available from the American Academy of Family Physicians.

ORDERING INFORMATION

Betamethasone sodium phosphate and acetate suspension (Celestone Soluspan 6 mg/mL, Schering-Plough, 2000 Galloping Hill Road, Kenilworth, NJ 07033; 908-298-4000)

1% lidocaine solution (Xylocaine, Astra U.S.A. Inc, 50 Otis Street, Westborough, MA 01581; 508-366-1100)

BIBLIOGRAPHY

Anderson LG. Aspirating and injecting the acutely painful joint. Emerg Med 1991; 23:77-94.

Brand C. Intra-articular and soft tissue injections. Austr Fam Physician 1990; 19:671-680.

Goss JA, Adams RF. Local injection of corticosteroids in rheumatic diseases. J Musculoskel Med 1993;10:83-92.

Gray RG, Gottlieb NL. Intra-articular corticosteroids: an updated assessment. Clin Orthop 1983;177:235-263.

Hollander JL. Arthrocentesis and intrasynovial therapy. In: McCarty DJ, ed. Arthritis. 9th ed. London: Henry Kimpton, 1979:402-414.

Leversee JH. Aspiration of joints and soft tissue injections. Prim Care 1986;13:579-599.

Owen DS, Irby R. Intra-articular and soft-tissue aspiration and injection. Clin Rheum Pract 1986;Mar/Apr/May:52-63.

Owen DS, Weiss JJ, Wilke WS. When to aspirate and inject joints. Pat Care 1990; 24:128-145.

Pando JA, Klippel JH. Arthrocentesis and corticosteroid injection: an illustrated guide to technique. Consultant 1996;36:2137-2148.

Stefanich RJ. Intraarticular corticosteroids in treatment of osteoarthritis. Orthop Rev 1986;15:27-33.

Schumacher HR. Arthrocentesis of the knee. Hosp Med 1997;33:60-64.

CHAPTER 22

Thoracentesis

Thoracentesis is a simple, commonly performed procedure that is used to evaluate or treat a collection of fluid in the pleural space. Diagnostic thoracentesis should be performed for nearly every patient who has a pleural effusion of unknown etiology; however, patients with confirmed congestive heart failure can appropriately be observed for a response to therapy. Therapeutic thoracentesis is performed to remove large volumes of fluid from patients with symptoms of respiratory distress.

It is estimated that 1.5 million Americans develop a pleural effusion each year. The recognition of a pleural effusion signals the presence of an abnormal physiologic state. The initial goal of diagnostic thoracentesis is to determine the cause for the abnormal production or clearance of fluid in the pleural space. The results of cytologic, hematologic, bacterial, and chemical analysis of the pleural fluid can be useful in management decisions.

Pleural effusions are classically divided into transudates and exudates. A transudate occurs when mechanical factors alter the formation or reabsorption of pleural fluid. Increased plasma oncotic pressure or pulmonary hydrostatic pressure can produce a transudate. The pleural surface usually is not involved by the primary pathologic process when a transudate exists.

An exudate results from inflammation or disease of the pleural surface. Causes of an exudate include infection, malignancy, pancreatitis, pulmonary infarction, or systemic lupus erythematosus (Tables 22.1 and 22.2). Historically, a pleural fluid protein level of 3.0 gm per dL was used to separate a transudate from an exudate; however, this dividing line failed to correctly characterize about 10% of effusions, especially the malignant exudates. A single chemical test is rarely 100% accurate in separating exudates from transudates.

An exudate can be correctly identified by the use of three markers in the pleural fluid. Exudates generally contain at least one of the following: a pleural fluid to serum protein ratio greater than 0.5, a pleural fluid lactic dehydrogenase (LDH) level greater than 200 IU, and a pleural fluid to serum LDH ratio greater than 0.6.

In addition to the above-mentioned tests that can distinguish an exudate from a transudate, there are other tests that can provide diagnostic clues. The appearance of the pleural fluid can help; a chylothorax, for example,

T‌ABLE 22.1. Causes of Transudates

Congestive heart failure
Cirrhosis of the liver
Nephrotic syndrome
Hypoalbuminemia
Peritoneal dialysis
Urinothorax
Atelectasis
Constrictive pericarditis
Superior vena cava obstruction

presents with milky fluid. An elevated white blood cell count can suggest infection, whereas low pH or low glucose can be seen in disease states such as an empyema. Bacterial, fungal, and Tb cultures can identify infectious sources. An elevated amylase can be associated with pancreatitis or esophageal rupture. Cytology studies can identify a malignant effusion.

Thoracentesis is relatively safe. The most common complication is pneumothorax, with an average incidence rate of 6 to 19%. Uncontrollable coughing during the procedure and the use of a large-bore needle (14-gauge) increase the likelihood of a postprocedure pneumothorax. Re-expansion pulmonary edema can develop in atelectatic lungs that have been collapsed for more than 7 days. To limit this complication and reduce postprocedure hypotension or shock, therapeutic thoracentesis should not remove more

T‌ABLE 22.2. Causes of Exudates

Parapneumonic effusions	Malignancy
Tuberculous pleurisy	Lymphoma
Pleural actinomycosis	Mesothelioma
Pleural nocardiosis	Aspergillosis
Pulmonary embolism	Uremia
Pulmonary infarction	Pancreatitis
Rheumatoid pleurisy	Liver abscess
Esophageal rupture	Sarcoidosis
Wegener's granulomatosis	Empyema
Meigs' syndrome	Chylothorax
Medications (e.g., amiodarone, nitrofurantoin, methotrexate)	Post MI injury
Sjögren's syndrome	Lupus pleuritis
Radiation pleuritis	Histoplasmosis
Postesophageal sclerotherapy	Benign asbestos
	Trapped lung

than 1.5 L of fluid at a time. Hemorrhage can develop in less than 2% of procedures and may necessitate thoracic surgery consultation if the bleeding is not controlled in 30 to 60 minutes.

METHODS AND MATERIALS

Patient Preparation

The patient and physician should be comfortably positioned for the procedure. An optimal position for the patient is to be seated, with the arms crossed, and the body resting on a support placed horizontally in front of the body. A sturdy, adjustable tray can be used for this support. Some authors also recommend a footstool to bring the upper legs to a horizontal position. The thorax should be as erect as possible.

Equipment

Sterile Thoracentesis Tray

The sterile, disposable thoracentesis tray is opened onto a Mayo stand, with the following items on the tray:

The thoracentesis catheter 18 cm (7 inch) long with a 14 gauge, 5.1 cm (2 inch) long needle attached

Catheter guard

60 mL lock tip syringe

25 gauge, 1.6 cm (⅝ inch) needle

22 gauge, 5.1 cm (2 inch) needle

3 way stopcock

5 mL syringe

Drainage tube and bag

3 prelabeled 10 mL specimen tubes with caps

2 swab sticks

3 gauze 3×3-inch sponges

Bandage for puncture site

Fenestrated drape with adhesive strips

Towel

5 mL of lidocaine HCl 1% (Xylocaine)

Povidone-iodine solution should be poured onto the tray into the plastic well. Sterile gloves must be supplied. A sterile hemostat can be added to the tray, if desired.

TABLE 22.3. **Estimates of Pleural Fluid on Chest X-ray**

Blunting of the costophrenic angle—100 to 150 mL
Half opacification of the hemithorax—1.0 to 1.5 L
Total opacification of the hemithorax—2.5 to 3.0 L

Adapted from Barbers R, Patel P. Thoracentesis made safe and simple. J Respir Dis 1994;5:841–851.

PROCEDURE DESCRIPTION

1. The preprocedure chest x-ray should be immediately available for review (Table 22.3). The fluid level on the lateral decubitus film should layer out to greater than 1 cm in thickness in order to perform the procedure safely in the office without ultrasound guidance.
2. The patient and physician should be comfortably positioned for the procedure. An optimal position for the patient is to be seated, with the arms crossed, and the body resting on a support placed horizontally in front of the body. A sturdy, adjustable tray can be used for this support. Some authors also recommend a footstool to bring the upper legs to a horizontal position. The thorax should be as erect as possible.
3. Because the physician is working behind the patient's back, each step of the procedure must be thoroughly explained to the patient. Proper patient information provides appropriate anticipation of the actions, invites cooperation, and reduces anxiety.
4. The level of effusion must be determined by percussion. The level lies at the point where the resonant percussion note (of the lungs) changes to a dull percussion note. The needle insertion site should be approximately one intercostal space below the level of effusion, at the upper portion of the rib, midway between the posterior axillary line and the paraspinal muscles (Fig. 22.1). Other authors advise insertion above the eighth rib, as low in the effusion as possible. Indent the insertion site with the fingernail to mark the skin.
5. Put on sterile gloves, and have the assistant open the thoracentesis tray, if used. Swab a large area around the insertion site with povidone-iodine solution, and center the sterile drape with the fenestration over the insertion site. The drape can be held with adhesive strips or tape applied to the upper edge.
6. Draw 5 to 10 mL of 1% lidocaine into the 10 mL syringe. A 25 gauge, ⅝ inch needle is used to create a skin wheal. A 22 gauge, ½ or 2 inch needle is placed on the syringe, and the needle is inserted until the tip touches the upper portion of the rib. Anesthetic is administered, the needle tip is slightly withdrawn, and is then redirected to just above the rib. The path of the needle tip is described as a "Z" insertion pattern. As the needle slowly advances, keep slight back pressure on the plunger

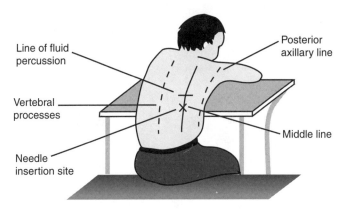

Line of fluid
percussion

Posterior
axillary line

Vertebral
processes

Middle line

Needle
insertion site

FIGURE 22.1. The patient is positioned with the arms crossed, leaning on an adjustable table. The insertion site for the needle will be the midpoint between the posterior axillary line and paraspinous muscles, one intercostal space below the percussed level of fluid.

to assess for fluid as you enter the pleural space. Stop every 2 mm, injecting lidocaine, until the pleural space is reached. Note the depth of the needle insertion, or place a hemostat on the needle, and then remove the needle from the patient.

7. For a diagnostic procedure, the 60 mL syringe is attached to the procedure needle. The thoracentesis tray uses a 7 inch intracatheter with a 14 gauge needle, although some physicians prefer to use a straight needle. A clamp can be placed on the needle to mark the depth needed to enter the pleural space (noted by the prior depth of insertion of the anesthesia needle). The needle enters the anesthetized skin, and the Z-track is used to advance the needle over the rib and into the pleural space (Fig. 22.2).

8. Remove the syringe and advance the catheter through the needle. Do not withdraw the catheter through the needle, as the tubing can be severed. The catheter guard can be placed to prevent damage to the catheter from the needle bevel. The syringe can be reattached, and pleural fluid aspirated. If a therapeutic procedure is performed, the stopcock can be attached to the drainage tubing and drainage bag. A maximum of 1.5 L is removed at one time.

9. The catheter is gently withdrawn at the end of the procedure. The insertion site can be gently rubbed, or pressure can be applied with gauze to ensure hemostasis and to confirm the absence of a fluid leak. A bandage is applied to the site.

10. Approximately 35 to 50 mL of fluid is necessary to complete the pleural fluid studies. The thoracentesis tray contains three 10 mL collection tubes. Fluid also can be sent to the laboratory in the procedure syringe.

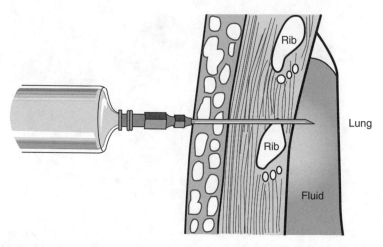

FIGURE 22.2. The needle is inserted just above the rib, avoiding the neurovascular bundle that lies just beneath the rib.

Some authors suggest that the following tests be performed on the pleural fluid of all patients undergoing thoracentesis: total protein, LDH, white blood cell count with differential, and glucose. A concomitant serum total protein, LDH, and glucose can be performed (usually immediately before the procedure). Other tests should be ordered based on clinical findings, or if the above tests confirm the presence of an exudate. Transudates are noninflammatory fluids with limited diagnostic possibilities.

11. Gram stain, KOH smear, AFB smear, and pleural fluid cultures can be performed when an infection is suspected with an exudative effusion. Some physicians will hold fluid in the laboratory until the presence of an exudate is confirmed. Pleural fluid cytology can be performed to exclude malignancy; lipid studies can be ordered on a milky supernatant; immunological studies can be performed for suspected lupus or rheumatoid pleuritis; and amylase can be performed for suspected pancreatitis, pancreatic pseudocyst, or esophageal rupture.

TABLE 22.4. CPT Codes

CPT Code	Description	1998 Total RVUs[a]	1998 Average 50% Fees in U.S.[b]
32000	Thoracentesis	2.52	$218

CPT only 1998 American Medical Association. All rights reserved.

[a] Department of Health and Human Services, Health Care Financing Administration. Medicare program: revisions to payment policies and adjustments to the relative value units (RVUs) under the physician fee schedule for calendar year 1998. Federal Register 42 CFR part 414. October 31, 1997;62(211):59103–59255.

[b] 1998 Physicians' Fee Reference. West Allis, WI: Yale Wasserman, DMD, Medical Publishers, 1998.

FOLLOW UP

See Tables 22.5-22.7.

TABLE 22.5. Information Obtained From Observation of Pleural Fluid

Bloody fluid: trauma, malignancy
White fluid: chyle, cholesterol, or empyema
Brown fluid: amebic liver abscess ruptures into the pleural space
Black fluid: aspergillus involvement of the pleura
Yellow-green fluid: rheumatoid pleuritis
Viscous effusion: increased hyaluronic acid from malignant mesothelioma
Debris in effusion: rheumatoid pleuritis
Putrid aroma: anaerobic empyema
Ammonia odor: urinothorax
Food particles in effusion: esophageal rupture

Adapted from Sahn SA. The pleura. Am Rev Respir Dis 1988;38:184–234.

TABLE 22.6. Transudative Pleural Effusions

Disease	Clinical Finding	Protein (g/dL)	LDH	Other Comments
Congestive heart failure	PND, rales, orthopnea, enlarged heart	0.6–3.8	10–190	
Cirrhosis	Ascites	PF/S ratio < 0.5	PF/S ratio < 0.6	Incidence is 6%
Peritoneal dialysis	Renal failure	< 1.0	< 100	Massive effusions may be encountered
Urinothorax	Urinary tract obstruction	< 1.0	< 175	Fluid has the odor of urine
Nephrotic syndrome	Edema	< 1.0	< 100	30% have pulmonary embolism
Atelectasis	Postoperative patients, lung cancer	PF/S ratio < 0.5	PF/S ratio < 0.6	

LDH, lactic dehydrogenase; PF/S, pleural fluid/serum.
Adapted from: Sahn SA. The pleura. Am Rev Respir Dis 1988;138:184–234.

TABLE 22.7. Exudative Pleural Effusions

Disease	Clinical Findings	Protein (g/dL)	LDH	Other Comments
Parapneumonic effusion	Pneumonia, turbid fluid	1.4–6.1	400 to > 1000	Complicated infections may require a chest tube
Tuberculosis	Cough, pleurisy, fever	> 4.0	< 700	Pleural biopsy, culture helpful
Aspergillosis	Cough, fever, weight loss, sputum prod.	PF/S ratio > 0.5	PF/S ratio > 0.6	Brown clumps, hyphae
Histoplasmosis	Cough, fever, malaise	4.1–5.7	200–425	Culture from pleural fluid
Viral infection	Acute chest pain following viral syndrome	3.2–4.9	PF/S ratio > 0.6	—
Mycoplasma infection	Cough, headache, myalgias	1.8–4.9	PF/S ratio > 0.6	Effusion resolves in days to weeks
Upper abdominal abscess	Fever, elevated WBC, abdominal pain	PF/S ratio > 0.5	PF/S ratio > 0.6	Effusion resolves with drainage
Esophageal perforation	Chest pain/fever following retching	PF/S ratio > 0.5	PF/S ratio > 0.6	Surgical closure preferred
Carcinoma	Cough, weight loss, ill appearing	1.5–8.0	300	Lung and breast most common
Lymphoma	Cough, dyspnea	PF/S ratio > 0.5	PF/S ratio > 0.6	Effusion poor prognostic sign
Mesothelioma	Males, asbestos exposure	3.5–5.5	36–600	Increased hyaluronic acid in fluid
Rheumatoid pleurisy	Males, moderate to severe arthritis	Up to 7.3	Frequently > 1000	Glucose < 30, pH 7.00
Lupus pleuritis	Known systemic lupus erythematosus, pleurisy, pleural rub	PF/S ratio > 0.5	PF/S ratio > 0.6	LE cells in the effusion
Post MI injury	Pleuritic pain, pericardial rub, fever	3.7	202	Effusion resolves spontaneously or with steroids
Sarcoidosis	Hilar adenopathy on chest x-ray	PF/S ratio > 0.5	PF/S ratio > 0.6	Effusion resolves spontaneously or with steroids
Pulmonary embolism	Pleuritic chest pain, tachypnea	Varies	Varies	Effusion reaches maximum volume by 72 hours
Pancreatitis	Abdominal pain, nausea, vomiting	PF/S ratio > 0.5	PF/S ratio > 0.6	Effusion resolves as pancreatitis resolves
Uremic effusion	Uremia > 1 year, fever, pleural rub	2.1–6.7	102–770	Effusion resolves with dialysis

LDH, lactic dehydrogenase; PF/S, pleural fluid/serum.
Adapted from: Sahn SA. The pleura. Am Rev Respir Dis 1988;138:184–234.

PROCEDURE PITFALLS/COMPLICATIONS

- *Air was aspirated during the procedure.* Aspiration of air during the procedure correlates with the development of a postprocedure pneumothorax. Excessive patient coughing during the procedure and the use of a large bore (14 gauge) needle can lead to this complication. Multiple attempts at thoracentesis and prior thoracic radiation therapy also is associated with developing a postprocedure pneumothorax.

- *The patient becomes hypoxemic following therapeutic removal of 1 L of pleural fluid.* Hypoxemia and unilateral pulmonary edema can develop following therapeutic thoracentesis. Half of all patients develop a decrease in PaO2, with some patients exhibiting a drop of 20 mm Hg; however, despite this decrease, many patients report relief of their dyspnea. The hypoxemia may relate to an immediate ventilation/perfusion mismatch in the area of expanded lung.

- *A vasovagal reaction occurs during the procedure.* Patients who develop a vasovagal reaction may become nauseated or presyncopal. If this reaction develops, the procedure should be immediately interrupted and the patient is put on the bed or floor as quickly as possible. Elevate the patient's feet to improve cerebral oxygen delivery. The sterile procedure field should be sacrificed for the long term safety of the patient.

- *Can the postprocedure chest x-ray be deferred following an uncomplicated procedure?* Despite the prior publication of guidelines that recommended postprocedure chest x-rays in most instances, many authors now question the value of this routine postprocedure examination. The chest x-ray should be performed when pneumothorax is clinically suspected, such as following the aspiration of air during the procedure. Occult pneumothoraxes are discovered by routine postprocedure chest x-ray, but since these often are not treated (unless the patient becomes symptomatic), the decision may be based on clinical findings.

- *Brisk bleeding is noted with needle insertion.* Bleeding complications can be reduced by choosing an insertion site along the superior aspect of the rib. Avoid the neurovascular bundle that courses along the inferior aspect of the rib. Minor bleeding is commonly observed following withdrawal of the needle, and usually ceases rapidly with direct pressure to the site.

PHYSICIAN TRAINING

Performing thoracentesis is relatively simple, and many physicians have initiated these procedures following the "see one, do one, teach one" methodology. Experience can help to select the proper needle insertion site and reduce the likelihood of a dry tap. Several articles have suggested that the complication rate from thoracentesis is lower among experienced physicians. It is recommended that physicians perform at least five supervised procedures before attempting thoracentesis unsupervised.

ORDERING INFORMATION

Thoracentesis tray (Baxter Pharmaseal Tray 4341A, Baxter Healthcare Corporation, Pharmaseal Division, Valencia, CA 91355-8900)

BIBLIOGRAPHY

Barbers R, Patel P. Thoracentesis made safe and simple. J Respir Dis 1994;15:841–851.

Collins TR, Sahn SA. Thoracentesis: clinical value, complications, technical problems, and patient experience. Chest 1987;91:817–822.

Doyle JJ, Hnatiuk OW, Torrington KG, Slade AR, Howard RS. Necessity of routine chest roentgenography after thoracentesis. Ann Intern Med 1996;124:816–820.

Johnson RL. Thoracentesis. In: Rakel RE, ed. Saunders manual of family practice. Philadelphia: WB Saunders, 1996:166–167.

Kuribayashi L. Pleural effusions. In: Rakel RE, ed. Saunders manual of family practice. Philadelphia: WB Saunders, 1996:164–165.

Light RW, MacGregor MI, Luchsinger PC, Ball WC. Pleural effusions: the diagnostic separation of transudates and exudates. Ann Intern Med 1972;77:507–513.

Meeker D. A stepwise approach to diagnostic and therapeutic thoracentesis. Modern Med 1993;61:62–71.

Roth BJ, O'Meara TF, Cragun WH. The serum-effusion albumin gradient in the evaluation of pleural effusions. Chest 1990;98:546–549.

Sahn SA, Good JT. Pleural fluid pH in malignant effusions: diagnostic, prognostic, and therapeutic implications. Ann Intern Med 1988;108:345–349.

Sahn SA. The pleura. Am Rev Respir Dis 1988;138:184–234.

APPENDIX A

●●

How to Decide Whether to Add a Procedure to Your Practice

This quick-reference guide presents a wide variety of procedures that can be included in your practice. The intent of the guide is not to make family physicians proficient in a new procedure, but to provide easy reference before performing the procedure. (Each chapter provides a general guideline for the number of procedures that should be done with a preceptor before beginning unsupervised procedures.)

But how do physicians decide whether to include a procedure in their practice? There are five major components to consider before adding a procedure: need for the procedure in the patient population, feasibility of performing the procedure in your office setting, cost of training for the physician and staff assistant(s), availability of a preceptor in your area, and economic implications for the practice. The following questions are issues that physicians should consider before deciding whether to perform a procedure.

NEED FOR THE PROCEDURE IN THE PATIENT POPULATION

- How many patients present to the practice with a complaint related to the procedure?
- How many referrals are made for the procedure to be performed?
- How many other physicians in the area perform the procedure? How convenient are they for your patient population?
- How acceptable will the procedure be to the patient population?
- Will the addition of the procedure to the practice have an impact on the diagnosis and management of the condition (i.e., allow you to provide a higher quality of care through improved diagnostic accuracy and timeliness of diagnosis and treatment)?

FEASIBILITY OF PERFORMING THE PROCEDURE IN THE OFFICE SETTING

- Do you have adequate space in the practice to perform the procedure?
- Does the space have appropriate set up for the equipment that the procedure requires?

- Is there a staff member (or members) available and willing to learn to assist with the procedure and care for the equipment properly?
- Is your schedule (and the schedule of the assistant) accommodating to the addition of the time that is needed to perform the procedure?
- By performing the procedure in the office, do you foresee that your patients will perceive a higher level of patient satisfaction (due to added convenience, comfort level with the physician, etc.)?

COST OF TRAINING FOR THE PHYSICIAN AND STAFF ASSISTANT(S)

- What is your current level of proficiency with related procedures or the procedure itself?
- How much training is necessary to become proficient in this procedure?
- Do you and the designated staff assistant have time to attend courses?
- What is the cost of training, and will it be recovered by performing the procedure?
- How much time and training is needed to maintain proficiency in the procedure?

AVAILABILITY OF A PRECEPTOR IN YOUR AREA

- Are there possible sources from which you can choose a preceptor (e.g., other family physicians who perform the procedure, residency faculty members, procedure course instructors, subspecialists)?
- Will the preceptor be available on a reasonably timely basis (allowing you to perform the procedure unsupervised in the time you have allotted for training)?
- Are the professional relations in your community strong enough so another physician would be willing to help you gain proficiency in the procedure?

ECONOMIC CONSIDERATIONS

- How much will the equipment for the procedure cost?
- How many procedures do you expect to perform each month?
- How much can you charge for the procedure, and what is the level of reimbursement for the procedure in your area?
- How long will it take for the equipment to pay for itself (see box on the next page)?
- Will the addition of the procedure benefit the financial position of the practice?

EASY AS ONE, TWO...

Here's one way to get a quick idea of whether a new procedure is worth your financial investment:

1. Calculate what you will earn doing the procedure:

(charge for the procedure) − (opportunity cost*) = revenue per procedure

2. Then, calculate how many procedures it will take to pay off the investment:

$$\frac{\text{cost of equipment}}{\text{revenue generated per procedure}} = \text{number of procedures needed}$$

---

*Opportunity cost is the revenue you normally generate in the time it would take to perform the new procedure.

Reprinted with permission from *Family Practice Management*, October 1993. Published by the American Academy of Family Physicians © 1993 AAFP.

INDEX

••

Page numbers in *italics* refer to figures; those followed by "t" refer to tables.

Acid laryngitis, 56
Actinic keratoses, 75
  cryosurgery for, 149
Acute diverticulitis, 41
Adenocarcinoma, 3
Adenoid hypertrophy, 57
Allergic disease, 56
Angiofibroma, 164
Anoscopy, 112
Arthrocentesis, 187
  indications for, 188*t*
Aspiration
  fine needle, for breast, 169-175
    CPT codes for, 174*t*
    equipment, 170
    follow up, 172, 173*t*
    patient preparation, 170
    physician training, 174
    procedure description, 170-171, *171, 172*
    procedure pitfalls/complications, 172-174
  of knee joint, 187-194
    contraindications for, 188*t*
    CPT codes for, 192*t*
    equipment, 189
    follow up, 191-193
    indications for, 188*t*
    patient preparation, 189
    physician training, 193
    procedure description, 189-191, *190, 191*
    procedure pitfalls/complications, 192-193
Aspiration pneumonia, 30
Association for Voluntary Surgical Contraception (AVSC), 147
Atypia, 3
  adenomatous, 11
Atypical squamous cells of undetermined significance (ASCUS), 3

Bacteremia, postprocedure, 20
Ballotment of the patella, 187
Barrett's esophasus, 29
Bartholin's cyst/abscess marsupialization, 81-86
  alternate procedures for, 81-82
  CPT codes for, 85*t*

differential diagnoses in, 82
equipment for, 82-83
follow up on, 84-85
patient preparation for, 82
physician training for, 86
procedure description, 83-84, *84*
procedure pitfalls/complications, 85-86
Bartholin's glands, 81
Basal cell carcinoma, 74-75, 164-165
Benign growths, 75
Biopsy. *See also* Open breast biopsy; Punch biopsy of the skin
  cervical, 4, 7-8, 10
  colpocopic, 132
  colposcopic, 11
  as component of EGD, 23
  endometrial, 15-21, 16*t*, *18, 19t*
  nondiagnostic, 30-31
  of soft lesion, 30
Blepharitis, chronic, 89
Blood taps, 48-49
Brain herniation, 48
Breast, fine-needle aspiration of, 169-175
  CPT codes for, 174*t*
  equipment, 170
  follow up, 172, 173*t*
  patient preparation, 170
  physician training, 174
  procedure description, 170-171, *171, 172*
  procedure pitfalls/complications, 172-174
Bursitis, 187

Cancer. *See* Carcinoma
Carcinoma
  basal cell, 164-165
  colon, 39
  colorectal, 35
  endometrial, 20
  laryngeal, 56
  squamous cell, 3, 165
Cellulitis, 192
Central nervous system malignancy, 43
Cerebrospinal fluid. *See also* Lumbar puncture
  characteristics of, in various conditions, 49*t*
  examination of, 43
Cervical biopsy, 4, 7-8, 10

209